WHICH WOLF WILL YOU FEED?

Also by Richard Sharratt

Productivity & Wellness: The Key to A Brighter Future

WHICH WOLF WILL YOU FEED?

Challenging the Stigma Around Men's Mental Health

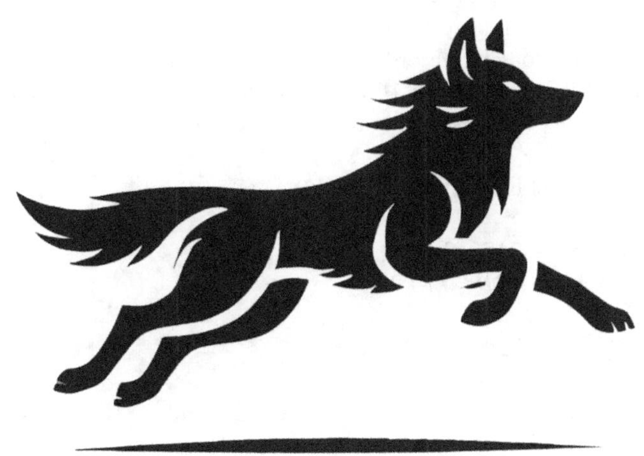

Richard Sharratt

With Foreword by
Willard Chesney

Contents

Foreword

Mental health is a topic that touches every life, but for some, the challenges are especially profound. Veterans and first responders—those who have dedicated themselves to service and protection—often find themselves facing battles unseen by others. The rigors of their professions, combined with the intense situations they encounter, place them at higher risk for mental health challenges that can be difficult to manage or even acknowledge.

Not only have I dealt with this myself, but I have seen it with many of my teammates. Many people struggling are taking their own lives, especially in the military and first responder community and this is unacceptable. I wish I had this book as a resource when I was still in the Navy to educate myself before things escalated to the point where I almost lost my own life.

Which Wolf seeks to shed light on these critical issues. It provides a comprehensive exploration of mental health, from its historical roots to the present-day understanding of symptoms, preventative measures, and treatments. But more importantly, it focuses on the unique needs of veterans and first responders—individuals who have faced the front lines of both visible and invisible battles.

By diving into the history of mental health, we can see how far we've come, but also how much work remains to be done. The knowledge of symptoms allows us to recognize the signs early, while preventatives and treatments offer hope and healing. Each chapter provides insight into the struggles faced by so many and offers guidance on the road to recovery, aiming to foster awareness, compassion, and support.

This book is not only a resource for veterans, first responders, their families, professionals and advocates who work with them but a resource and guidebook for anyone struggling. Everyone will deal with situations in life that will affect their mental health in some capacity, but everybody's journey in life is different and their struggles will not be the same. Let this be a resource to help either yourself or someone you care about.

To those who serve or have served: this book is for you and the families that support them. May it remind you that you are not alone, that healing is possible, and that help is always within reach. It is my hope that it will serve as a beacon of understanding and a call to action—because acknowledging and addressing mental health is not just a personal journey; it's a societal responsibility.

You are never out of the fight.

—Willard Chesney, US Navy SEAL (Ret.)

WHICH WOLF WILL YOU FEED?

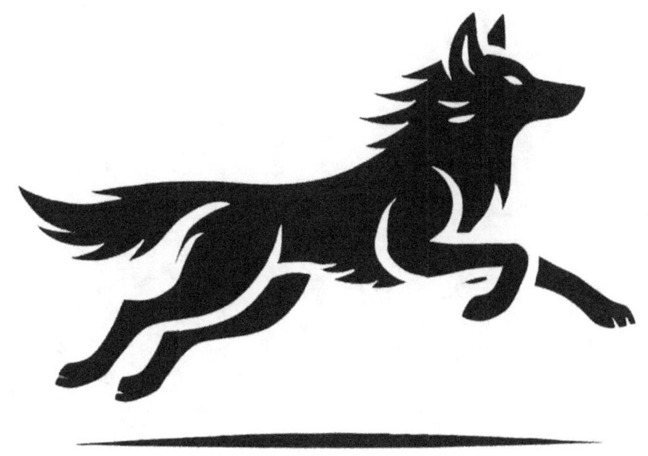

Chapter 1

The Cherokee Legend of the Two Wolves
Which Wolf Will You Feed?

Introduction to the Cherokee Legend

The Cherokee legend of the two wolves is a powerful and timeless story that has been passed down through generations. It serves as a profound metaphor for the inner struggles we all face and the choices we make in our daily lives. This chapter explores the legend, its meanings, and how it can be applied to help men grow and succeed. Additionally, it highlights how the story is pivotal to the work that the charity MENtality Matters does with men, veterans and first responders throughout the United States and the rest of the world.

The Legend of the Two Wolves

The Story

The story of the two wolves is often told as follows:

An old Cherokee is teaching his grandson about life. "A fight is going on inside me," he said to the boy.

"It is a terrible fight, and it is between two wolves. One is evil—he is anger, envy, sorrow, regret, greed, arrogance, self-pity, guilt, resentment, inferiority, lies, false pride, superiority, and ego."

He continued, "The other is good—he is joy, peace, love, hope, serenity, humility, kindness, benevolence, empathy, generosity, truth, compassion, and faith. The same fight is going on inside you—and inside every other person, too."

The grandson thought about it for a minute and then asked his grandfather, "Which wolf will win?"

The old Cherokee simply replied, "The one you feed."

Interpreting the Legend

Inner Conflict

The legend of the two wolves represents the inner conflict that exists within every individual. We all have impulses, thoughts, and emotions that can lead us down different paths. The "evil" wolf symbolizes negative traits and destructive behaviors, while the "good" wolf embodies positive attributes and constructive actions.

This internal battle is universal, transcending cultures and backgrounds. It is a fundamental aspect of the human experience, and understanding this can help individuals recognize the power of their choices in shaping their lives. The story underscores that everyone, regardless of their background or experiences, grapples with these conflicting impulses.

The Power of Choice

The key message of the legend is the power of choice. It emphasizes that we have the agency to choose which wolf to feed—whether we nurture positive qualities or give in to negative tendencies. This concept is empowering because it places responsibility and control in the hands of the individual.

Every decision we make, no matter how small, contributes to which wolf grows stronger. By consistently making choices that align with our values and aspirations, we can cultivate a life filled with positivity and purpose. This understanding fosters a sense of personal accountability and encourages proactive decision-making.

Applying the Legend to Men's Growth and Success

Self-Awareness and Reflection

The first step in applying the legend is developing self-awareness. Men need to recognize the internal struggle and identify the thoughts and behaviors associated with each wolf. Reflection and mindfulness practices can help individuals become more attuned to their inner dialogue and emotional responses.

1. **Journaling:** Keeping a journal can help men track their thoughts and emotions, providing insight into patterns and triggers. Writing about daily experiences can reveal which wolf they are feeding

and help them make conscious adjustments. For example, noting instances of anger or kindness can highlight areas for growth and improvement.

2. **Mindfulness Meditation:** Practicing mindfulness meditation allows men to observe their thoughts without judgment. This awareness can create a space between impulse and action, enabling better decision-making. Techniques such as focused breathing, body scans, and guided imagery can enhance mindfulness practices.

3. **Therapeutic Reflection:** Engaging in reflective practices during therapy sessions can help men explore their inner conflicts. Therapists can guide clients through exercises that examine their choices and the underlying motivations behind them, fostering deeper self-understanding.

Making Positive Choices

Once self-awareness is established, the focus shifts to making positive choices. This involves consciously choosing actions that feed the good wolf and align with personal values and goals.

1. **Setting Goals:** Clear, achievable goals provide direction and purpose. Men can set specific targets for personal growth, such as improving relationships, advancing in their careers, or enhancing physical health. Setting both short-term and long-term goals can provide a roadmap for continuous improvement.

2. **Practicing Gratitude:** Gratitude practices, such as listing things they are thankful for each day, can shift focus from negative to positive aspects of life. This simple habit can significantly enhance overall well-being. Research has shown that gratitude can improve mood, increase resilience, and foster a positive outlook.

3. **Engaging in Positive Activities:** Participating in activities that promote joy, peace, and connection can help feed the good wolf. This might include hobbies, volunteer work, or spending time with loved ones. Activities such as exercise, creative pursuits, and social engagement are particularly beneficial for mental health.

4. **Mindful Consumption of Media:** Being mindful of the media one consumes is also important. Choosing to engage with positive, uplifting content rather than negative or sensationalist news can

influence one's mindset and emotions. Curating a social media feed to include inspiring and supportive content can also make a significant difference.

Overcoming Challenges

Feeding the good wolf is not always easy, especially in the face of challenges and adversity. Men must develop resilience and coping strategies to maintain their focus on positive growth.

1. **Building a Support Network:** Surrounding oneself with supportive and positive individuals can provide encouragement and accountability. This network can include friends, family, mentors, or support groups. Engaging with a community of like-minded individuals can reinforce positive behaviors and attitudes.

2. **Seeking Professional Help:** When facing significant challenges, professional help from therapists or counselors can provide valuable guidance and support. Mental health professionals can help men develop strategies to manage stress, anxiety, and other issues. Therapy can offer a safe space to explore and address deep-seated issues and emotions.

3. **Learning from Setbacks:** Setbacks are inevitable, but they do not define one's journey. Men can view challenges as opportunities for learning and growth, reinforcing their commitment to feeding the good wolf. Reflecting on setbacks and understanding the lessons they offer can build resilience and perseverance.

4. **Developing Coping Mechanisms:** Effective coping mechanisms, such as exercise, relaxation techniques, and creative expression, can help manage stress and negative emotions. These strategies can provide healthy outlets for processing emotions and maintaining mental balance.

5. **Engaging in Community Service:** Helping others through volunteer work or community service can foster a sense of purpose and connection. Acts of kindness and service not only benefit others but also reinforce positive self-identity and fulfilment.

MENtality Matters and the Legend of the Two Wolves

The Charity's Mission

MENtality Matters is dedicated to supporting men's mental health and honoring our veteran and first responder heroes. The organization provides resources, education, and support to help men navigate mental health challenges and access necessary care. The legend of the two wolves is central to the charity's approach, emphasizing the power of choice and personal responsibility in mental health and well-being.

While this book will be focusing on men's and veterans' mental health, the strategies can be employed within any industry, including first responders.

Programs and Initiatives

MENtality Matters incorporates the principles of the two wolves legend into its programs and initiatives, helping men and veterans make positive choices and build fulfilling lives.

1. **Warriors Haven Program:** This flagship program offers veterans a safe and supportive environment to engage in therapeutic activities, receive support, and connect with peers. The retreat uses the legend of the two wolves to teach veterans about the importance of nurturing positive qualities and making empowering choices. Activities such as guided reflections, group discussions, and individual coaching sessions are all designed to reinforce these principles.

2. **Warriors Workshops:** MENtality Matters conducts workshops that focus on self-awareness, goal setting, and resilience. These workshops draw on the lessons of the two wolves legend to help men understand the impact of their choices and develop strategies for personal growth. Interactive exercises, role-playing scenarios, and practical tools are used to engage participants and facilitate learning.

3. **Warriors Ruck/Support Groups:** The charity facilitates peer support groups where men can share their experiences, offer support, and hold each other accountable. The story of the two wolves serves as a guiding principle in these groups, encouraging

men to support each other in feeding the good wolf. Regular meetings, peer mentorship programs, and community-building activities are integral parts of these groups.

4. **Mentorship Programs:** MENtality Matters also runs mentorship programs that pair experienced mentors with men seeking guidance and support. Mentors use the two wolves legend to help mentees reflect on their choices and develop positive habits. This relationship fosters personal growth, accountability, and mutual respect.

5. **Resource Distribution:** The charity provides educational materials, such as booklets and online resources, that explain the two wolves legend and offer practical advice for feeding the good wolf. These resources are distributed through workshops, retreats, and the charity's website.

Impact on Men's Mental Health

The application of the two wolves legend has had a profound impact on the men and veterans served by MENtality Matters. By fostering self-awareness, positive decision-making, and resilience, the charity helps individuals improve their mental health and overall quality of life.

1. **Personal Transformations:** Many participants report significant improvements in their mental health and well-being. They describe feeling more in control of their lives and better equipped to handle challenges. Success stories highlight how individuals have overcome adversity, rebuilt relationships, and found new purpose.

2. **Community and Connection:** The programs foster a sense of community and connection, reducing feelings of isolation and promoting a supportive network of peers. Participants often form lasting friendships and support networks that extend beyond the programs.

3. **Long-Term Success:** By internalizing the lessons of the two wolves legend, participants are better able to maintain positive habits and continue their personal growth journey long after completing the programs. Follow-up support and ongoing engagement with MENtality Matters ensure that participants remain connected and supported.

4. **Feedback and Testimonials:** Feedback from participants consistently highlights the transformative impact of the programs. Testimonials often mention the profound influence of the two wolves legend in helping individuals make positive changes in their lives.

5. **Measurable Outcomes:** The charity tracks measurable outcomes, such as reductions in symptoms of depression and anxiety, increased resilience, and improved overall well-being. These metrics demonstrate the effectiveness of the programs and the importance of the two wolves legend in fostering positive change.

Integrating the Legend into Daily Life

Practical Steps for Men

Integrating the lessons of the two wolves legend into daily life involves making conscious choices that reinforce positive behaviors and attitudes.

1. **Daily Reflection:** Take a few minutes each day to reflect on the choices made and the emotions experienced. Consider which wolf was fed and how future choices can align more closely with personal values.

2. **Setting Intentions:** Start each day by setting positive intentions. Decide what qualities to nurture and what actions to take to feed the good wolf. This practice can provide focus and motivation throughout the day.

3. **Mindful Decision-Making:** Pause before making decisions, especially in moments of stress or conflict. Consider the potential impact of the decision on personal well-being and relationships. Choose actions that align with feeding the good wolf.

4. **Positive Affirmations:** Use positive affirmations to reinforce self-worth and encourage positive thinking. Statements such as "I am capable," "I choose kindness," and "I am in control of my choices" can help strengthen the good wolf.

5. **Seeking Support:** Don't hesitate to seek support from friends, family, or professionals. Sharing experiences and seeking advice can provide valuable perspectives and encouragement.

Applying the Legend in Professional Settings

The lessons of the two wolves legend can also be applied in professional settings to enhance workplace culture and personal career growth.

1. **Leadership and Management:** Leaders can use the legend to promote positive values and behaviors within their teams. Encouraging open communication, empathy, and collaboration can create a supportive and productive work environment.

2. **Conflict Resolution:** The legend provides a framework for resolving conflicts by focusing on positive outcomes and mutual respect. Encouraging individuals to reflect on their choices and prioritize constructive behaviors can help resolve disputes effectively.

3. **Professional Development:** Individuals can use the legend to guide their professional development. Setting goals, seeking mentorship, and engaging in continuous learning are all ways to feed the good wolf in a career context.

4. **Team Building:** Incorporating the legend into team-building activities can foster a sense of unity and shared purpose. Discussing the story and its implications can help team members understand each other better and work more cohesively.

The Cherokee legend of the two wolves offers a powerful framework for understanding and addressing the inner struggles we all face. By recognizing the internal battle between negative and positive impulses and making conscious choices to feed the good wolf, men can achieve personal growth and success.

MENtality Matters uses this legend as a cornerstone of its work, helping men, veterans, and first responders throughout the USA develop self-awareness, make positive choices, and build fulfilling lives. The legend's message of empowerment and personal responsibility is pivotal to the charity's mission and the impact it has on the lives of those it serves.

By embracing the lessons of the two wolves, men can take control of their mental health and well-being, fostering resilience, growth, and success in all areas of life. The principles of the legend can be applied in personal, professional, and community contexts, offering a versatile and enduring guide for positive living.

The journey of self-improvement and mental well-being is ongoing, and the legend of the two wolves provides a timeless and accessible tool for navigating this path. It reminds us that we have the power to shape our lives through our choices and that nurturing the positive aspects of our nature can lead to a more fulfilling and meaningful existence.

The work of MENtality Matters demonstrates the profound impact that this legend can have when integrated into structured support programs. By continuing to promote these principles, we can create a society that values mental health, supports personal growth, and honors the contributions and sacrifices of our veterans and first responders.

The legend of the two wolves is not just a story but a call to action. It challenges us to reflect on our choices, embrace our potential, and strive for a life that is rich in joy, peace, and purpose. Whether through individual efforts or collective initiatives like those of MENtality Matters, we can all contribute to a world where the good wolf thrives.

Chapter 2

Historical Overview of Mental Health in the USA

Introduction to Historical Context

Understanding the history of mental health in the United States is crucial for comprehending the current landscape and the challenges faced today. This chapter delves into the evolution of mental health perceptions, treatments, and policies, providing a comprehensive overview from early history to the present day. By tracing this evolution, we can better appreciate the progress made and the obstacles that remain in addressing mental health issues.

Mental health has always been a vital component of overall well-being, yet its recognition and treatment have evolved significantly over the centuries. From ancient misconceptions and harsh treatments to modern understandings and therapies, the journey of mental health care in America reflects broader societal changes and advancements in medical science. This chapter will explore the historical milestones, key figures, and pivotal moments that have shaped the current mental health landscape.

Early Perceptions and Treatments:

Ancient and Colonial Era Views on Mental Health

In ancient times, mental health issues were often misunderstood and attributed to supernatural causes. People with mental illnesses were thought to be possessed by spirits or demons, and treatments were aimed at expelling these forces. Practices such as trepanning (drilling holes in the skull) were common, reflecting the belief that mental illness resulted from evil spirits trapped in the head.

During the colonial era in America, mental illness was still largely viewed through a religious or moral lens. Those with mental health issues were often seen as sinners or morally weak individuals. Treatments were rudimentary and included confinement, physical restraints, and even exorcisms. There

11

was little understanding of mental illness as a medical condition, and those affected were frequently ostracized or hidden away.

Early Treatments and Institutions

The establishment of early asylums in the 18th and early 19th centuries marked the beginning of institutional care for the mentally ill. However, these institutions were far from humane. Conditions were often deplorable, and treatments were harsh. Patients were subjected to isolation, restraints, and other inhumane practices.

One of the earliest institutions, the Pennsylvania Hospital, established in 1751, included one of the first wards for the mentally ill in America. Despite its pioneering status, conditions were far from ideal, and treatments were primitive. Patients were often kept in chains or confined to small, dark rooms, with little to no therapeutic intervention.

Another early institution, Williamsburg's Public Hospital, opened in 1773 in Virginia. It was the first public institution in America dedicated solely to the care of the mentally ill. However, treatments were often harsh, focusing more on containment than on cure. Patients were subjected to physical restraints and isolation, with little regard for their dignity or well-being.

The early asylums reflected a broader societal view that saw mental illness as something to be hidden and controlled rather than understood and treated. These institutions operated more like prisons than hospitals, with the primary goal of keeping patients away from the general population.

19th Century Developments:

Introduction of More Humane Treatment Approaches

The 19th century saw the beginning of a shift towards more humane treatment of the mentally ill. The "moral treatment" movement emerged, emphasizing kindness, respect, and improved living conditions for patients.

Philippe Pinel, a French physician, is often credited with pioneering the moral treatment approach. He advocated for the unchaining of patients and the provision of more humane care. Pinel's work in France inspired similar reforms in the United States, where mental health care began to focus more on the well-being and dignity of patients.

Dorothea Dix, an American social reformer, conducted extensive research and advocacy, leading to significant improvements in the care of the mentally ill. Her efforts resulted in the establishment of more than 30 state mental hospitals in the United States. Dix's work highlighted the need for better conditions and more compassionate care, marking a significant step forward in mental health treatment.

The moral treatment movement emphasized the importance of a supportive and therapeutic environment. Patients were encouraged to engage in activities, interact with others, and participate in their own care. This approach represented a significant departure from the harsh and punitive methods of the past, recognizing the humanity and potential for recovery in every patient.

Key Figures and Contributions

Several key figures played crucial roles in advancing mental health care during the 19th century:

—**Benjamin Rush:** Often referred to as the "father of American psychiatry," Rush was a signatory of the Declaration of Independence and a pioneering figure in the treatment of mental illness. He promoted the idea that mental illness was a disease of the mind and should be treated with compassion and medical care. Rush's work laid the foundation for modern psychiatric practices, and his advocacy for humane treatment helped shift societal attitudes towards mental illness.

—**Clifford Beers:** A former mental patient, Beers became an advocate for mental health reform. His autobiography, "A Mind That Found Itself," highlighted the abuses in mental institutions and spurred the mental hygiene movement. Beers' work led to the establishment of organizations dedicated to improving mental health care and reducing stigma.

—**Elizabeth Packard:** An advocate for the rights of the mentally ill, Packard fought against unjust institutionalization practices. Her own experiences of being wrongfully committed by her husband led her to campaign for legal reforms and greater protections for mental health patients.

These individuals and others like them played vital roles in changing public perceptions and improving the treatment of mental health issues. Their contributions laid the groundwork for further advancements in the 20th century.

20th Century Advances:

Emergence of Psychoanalysis and Psychotherapy

The early 20th century saw significant advancements in the understanding and treatment of mental health issues. Sigmund Freud's theories of psychoanalysis introduced the concept of exploring unconscious thoughts and childhood experiences to treat mental illness. Freud's work laid the foundation for various forms of psychotherapy, which became more widespread and accepted as legitimate treatments for mental health issues.

Psychoanalysis emphasized the importance of understanding the underlying psychological causes of mental illness. This approach represented a significant shift from earlier views that focused primarily on physical symptoms and treatments. Freud's theories, while controversial, opened the door to new ways of thinking about and treating mental health conditions.

The development of other therapeutic approaches, such as behaviorism and humanistic psychology, further expanded the range of treatment options available. Behaviorism, led by figures like John B. Watson and B.F. Skinner, focused on the idea that behaviors could be learned and unlearned. This led to the development of various therapeutic techniques aimed at modifying behavior.

Humanistic psychology, championed by Carl Rogers and Abraham Maslow, emphasized the importance of individual potential and self-actualization. This approach focused on creating a supportive and empathetic therapeutic environment, encouraging patients to explore their feelings and experiences.

Establishment of Mental Health Policies and Organizations

The mid-20th century marked significant progress in mental health care with the establishment of key organizations and policies. The National Institute of Mental Health (NIMH), established in 1949, played a crucial role in funding research, promoting education, and improving treatments for mental health conditions. The NIMH's efforts helped to advance the understanding of mental health issues and support the development of more effective treatments.

The Community Mental Health Act of 1963, signed by President John F. Kennedy, aimed to deinstitutionalize mental health care and provide community-based services. This legislation was a response to the growing recognition that large institutions were often inadequate and inhumane. The act sought to shift the focus of mental health care to local communities, providing more accessible and integrated services.

While well-intentioned, the implementation of the Community Mental Health Act faced significant challenges. Inadequate funding, lack of infrastructure, and insufficient community resources hampered the transition from institutional care to community-based services. Many individuals who were released from institutions struggled to find the support they needed, leading to an increase in homelessness and other social issues.

Despite these challenges, the act represented a significant step forward in the recognition of mental health as a public health issue. It underscored the importance of providing comprehensive care that addresses both mental and physical health needs.

Advances in Psychiatric Medications and Treatments

The development of psychiatric medications revolutionized the treatment of mental health conditions. The introduction of antipsychotic medications in the 1950s provided effective treatment for schizophrenia and other severe mental illnesses. These medications helped to manage symptoms and improve the quality of life for many individuals.

The development of antidepressants and mood stabilizers in the latter half of the 20th century offered new hope for those suffering from depression and bipolar disorder. Medications like selective serotonin reuptake inhibitors (SSRIs) became widely used, providing effective relief for many patients.

Advances in psychiatric medications were accompanied by improvements in other forms of treatment, including various types of psychotherapy. Cognitive-behavioral therapy (CBT), developed in the 1960s, emerged as an effective treatment for a range of mental health conditions. CBT focuses on identifying and changing negative thought patterns and behaviors, helping patients develop healthier coping strategies.

The combination of medication and therapy provided a more comprehensive approach to mental health care, addressing both biological and psychological aspects of mental illness. These advancements represented significant progress in the field, offering new possibilities for treatment and recovery.

Modern Era:

Integration of Mental Health Care into General Health Care

In recent decades, there has been a growing recognition of the importance of integrating mental health care into general health care systems. This approach emphasizes a holistic understanding of health, recognizing the interconnection between physical and mental well-being.

Holistic approaches to mental health care focus on treating the whole person, addressing both physical and mental health needs. This includes considering factors such as lifestyle, social support, and environmental influences. Integrating mental health care into primary care settings helps to ensure that individuals receive comprehensive and coordinated care.

Collaborative care models have become increasingly common, involving primary care providers, mental health specialists, and other professionals working together to provide comprehensive care. These models aim to improve access to mental health services, reduce stigma, and ensure that patients receive timely and appropriate treatment.

Efforts to integrate mental health care into general health care systems have also focused on addressing disparities in access to care. Initiatives aimed at improving mental health care for underserved populations, including racial and ethnic minorities, rural communities, and low-income individuals, are critical to ensuring equitable access to services.

Current State of Mental Health Care and Ongoing Challenges

Despite the progress made, significant challenges remain in addressing mental health issues in the United States. Stigma continues to be a major barrier to seeking treatment, with many individuals reluctant to discuss their mental health struggles due to fear of judgment or discrimination. Efforts to reduce stigma include public awareness campaigns, education initiatives, and advocacy work.

Access to care remains a significant issue, particularly for individuals in rural or underserved areas. Many areas face a shortage of mental health professionals, and financial constraints and insurance limitations can further restrict access to services. Addressing these barriers requires targeted efforts to increase the availability of mental health services and ensure that they are affordable and accessible to all.

Disparities in treatment persist, with racial, ethnic, and socioeconomic differences in access to care and treatment outcomes. These disparities highlight the need for culturally competent care and targeted interventions to ensure that all individuals receive equitable and effective mental health care.

The COVID-19 pandemic has further highlighted the importance of robust mental health care systems. The pandemic has led to increased rates of anxiety, depression, and other mental health issues, underscoring the need for accessible and comprehensive mental health services. The crisis has also emphasized the importance of addressing the social determinants of health, including economic stability, social support, and access to care.

The history of mental health care in the United States reflects a journey from misunderstanding and mistreatment to greater awareness and more effective treatments. While substantial progress has been made, ongoing efforts are needed to ensure that mental health care is accessible, compassionate, and effective for all. This historical context sets the stage for understanding the current mental health crisis among men and military veterans, which will be explored in the following chapters.

By examining the past, we can better understand the challenges and opportunities that lie ahead. The following chapters will delve into the specific issues facing men and military veterans, exploring the current mental health crisis and the efforts to address it. Through a comprehensive understanding of history and present-day challenges, we can work towards a future where mental health care is accessible, effective, and free from stigma.

Chapter 3

Historical Overview of Military and Veteran Mental Health

Introduction to Military Mental Health History

Understanding the history of mental health within the military context is essential for grasping the unique challenges faced by service members and veterans. The experiences of soldiers in various conflicts have shaped the understanding and treatment of mental health issues. This chapter delves into the evolution of military mental health, tracing key developments and recognizing the strides made in care and treatment.

The mental health of military personnel has long been a critical concern, as the stresses of combat and military life can have profound effects on psychological well-being. Over time, the understanding and approach to military mental health have evolved significantly, reflecting broader changes in societal attitudes, medical knowledge, and military practices.

Mental Health in Early Military History:

Mental Health During the Revolutionary War and Civil War

During the Revolutionary War and Civil War, mental health issues among soldiers were often overlooked or misunderstood. Soldiers experiencing psychological distress were frequently viewed as weak or lacking in moral fiber. There was little recognition of the impact of combat stress, and mental health issues were rarely addressed in a meaningful way.

The harsh conditions of warfare, combined with limited medical knowledge, meant that many soldiers suffering from mental health issues were left untreated. Those exhibiting signs of distress were often subjected to disciplinary action or deemed unfit for duty. The lack of understanding and appropriate care resulted in significant suffering for many soldiers.

For example, during the Civil War, the term "nostalgia" was used to describe what we would now recognize as depression. Soldiers who experienced severe homesickness, anxiety, and depression were often dismissed as malingerers. Treatments were limited and largely ineffective, and many soldiers faced their struggles alone.

While the physical toll of the Civil War was immense, the psychological toll was also significant. The war's brutality, combined with the primitive medical care available at the time, left many soldiers with deep psychological scars. The lack of formal recognition and treatment for these issues meant that many soldiers suffered in silence.

Early Recognition of War-Related Psychological Issues

Despite the lack of formal recognition, there were instances where the psychological impact of warfare was acknowledged. Terms like "nostalgia" (now understood as depression) and "irritable heart" (an early descriptor of anxiety) were used to describe soldiers' conditions. However, these terms were not widely accepted, and treatment options remained limited.

The early recognition of these issues laid the groundwork for future advancements in understanding and addressing the mental health needs of soldiers. As military conflicts continued, the need for better mental health care became increasingly evident. These early observations were crucial in highlighting the psychological toll of combat and the necessity for more comprehensive care.

During the Civil War, medical practitioners like Dr. Jacob Mendez Da Costa began to study the symptoms of what he termed "irritable heart," now known as Da Costa's syndrome. This condition, characterized by palpitations, chest pain, and fatigue, was recognized as a form of combat-related anxiety. While treatments remained rudimentary, the identification of such conditions represented an important step forward.

World Wars and Mental Health Awareness:

"Shell Shock" in World War I

World War I marked a significant turning point in the recognition of combat-related psychological issues. The term "shell shock" was coined to describe the symptoms exhibited by soldiers exposed to the intense and sustained artillery bombardments of trench warfare. Symptoms included severe anxiety, tremors, nightmares, and an inability to function.

The widespread occurrence of shell shock among soldiers prompted military and medical authorities to take the condition seriously. Although initial treatment efforts were rudimentary and often ineffective, the recognition of shell shock represented an important step toward understanding the psychological impact of war.

During World War I, shell shock was often misunderstood and misdiagnosed. Some medical professionals believed it was caused by physical damage to the brain from shell explosions, while others thought it was a sign of cowardice or moral weakness. Treatments varied widely, from rest and relaxation to disciplinary measures. The lack of a unified approach reflected the limited understanding of the condition.

As the war progressed, the scale of the shell shock problem became impossible to ignore. Military hospitals in Europe and the United States were filled with soldiers exhibiting symptoms of severe psychological distress. Efforts to treat these soldiers varied widely, with some receiving compassionate care while others faced harsh treatment or even punishment.

The work of pioneering psychiatrists like W.H.R. Rivers in the United Kingdom began to shed light on the psychological causes of shell shock. Rivers and his colleagues advocated for more humane and effective treatments, including psychotherapy and rest. Their work laid the foundation for future advancements in military mental health care.

Advances in Understanding and Treatment During World War II

World War II saw further advancements in the understanding and treatment of combat-related mental health issues. The term "combat fatigue" was used to describe psychological distress resulting from prolonged exposure to combat. The U.S. military implemented screening processes to identify individuals at risk of developing combat fatigue and established rest and rehabilitation programs.

The work of psychiatrists like William Menninger and Roy Grinker contributed to a better understanding of combat-related mental health issues. Their research and clinical work helped to refine treatment approaches and improve outcomes for affected soldiers. The establishment of military psychiatric units and the use of therapeutic techniques marked significant progress in addressing mental health needs.

World War II also saw the introduction of more systematic and organized approaches to mental health care within the military. The military developed specialized training programs for medical personnel to better identify and treat psychological issues. These efforts were crucial in reducing the stigma associated with mental health problems and providing more effective care.

The understanding of combat fatigue evolved throughout the war, with a growing recognition that psychological stress could affect any soldier, regardless of their courage or resilience. This shift in perspective led to more compassionate and effective treatments, including rest periods, counseling, and rehabilitation programs.

The establishment of the Menninger Clinic in Kansas by Dr. William Menninger and his brother Karl provided a model for comprehensive psychiatric care. The clinic became a leading center for the treatment of combat-related mental health issues, emphasizing the importance of early intervention and holistic care.

Vietnam War and PTSD Recognition:

Mental Health Challenges Faced by Vietnam Veterans

The Vietnam War presented unique mental health challenges for service members. The nature of the conflict, combined with the political and social climate in the United States, contributed to high levels of psychological distress among returning veterans. Issues such as drug addiction, depression, and anxiety were prevalent, but there was limited support available.

Vietnam veterans faced significant challenges in reintegrating into civilian life. The lack of public support for the war, combined with negative perceptions of veterans, exacerbated their struggles. Many veterans turned to substance abuse as a coping mechanism, and rates of homelessness and unemployment were high among this population.

The psychological impact of the Vietnam War was profound. Veterans experienced high levels of trauma due to the nature of the conflict, which involved guerrilla warfare, ambushes, and constant threat. The use of chemical agents like Agent Orange added to the physical and psychological toll. The anti-war sentiment and societal division back home further alienated veterans, making it difficult for them to receive the support and recognition they needed.

The experiences of Vietnam veterans highlighted the need for a more comprehensive understanding of combat-related mental health issues. The war's psychological toll led to increased research and advocacy, paving the way for significant advancements in mental health care for veterans.

Emergence of PTSD as a Recognized Condition

One of the most significant developments during the post-Vietnam era was the recognition of Post-Traumatic Stress Disorder (PTSD) as a distinct condition. The experiences of Vietnam veterans played a crucial role in the formal inclusion of PTSD in the Diagnostic and Statistical Manual of Mental Disorders (DSM-III) in 1980. This recognition marked a significant advancement in understanding and treating trauma-related mental health issues.

The establishment of PTSD as a recognized condition led to increased research and the development of specialized treatment approaches. This period also saw the growth of veteran advocacy groups, which played a key role in raising awareness and pushing for better mental health care for veterans.

The recognition of PTSD was a critical milestone in mental health care, as it acknowledged the long-term psychological impact of combat and other traumatic experiences. The development of evidence-based treatments, such as Cognitive Behavioral Therapy (CBT) and Eye Movement Desensitization and Reprocessing (EMDR), provided new tools for addressing PTSD and improving outcomes for affected individuals.

The inclusion of PTSD in the DSM-III was a result of extensive research and advocacy by mental health professionals and veterans' organizations. The work of psychiatrists like Dr. Robert Jay Lifton and Dr. Jonathan Shay was instrumental in highlighting the psychological impact of combat and advocating for the recognition of PTSD.

The formal recognition of PTSD brought much-needed attention to the mental health needs of veterans. It also led to the establishment of specialized programs within the Department of Veterans Affairs (VA) to provide targeted care and support for veterans with PTSD.

Recent Conflicts and Advances in Mental Health Care:

Mental Health Issues in the Gulf War, Iraq, and Afghanistan

Recent conflicts, including the Gulf War, Iraq, and Afghanistan, have further highlighted the mental health challenges faced by military personnel. Issues such as PTSD, depression, and traumatic brain injury (TBI) have been prevalent among service members. The nature of modern warfare, with its prolonged deployments and exposure to improvised explosive devices (IEDs), has contributed to these challenges.

The Department of Defense (DoD) and the Department of Veterans Affairs (VA) have implemented various programs to address the mental health needs of service members and veterans. These programs include screening, early intervention, and evidence-based treatments designed to support mental health and well-being.

One of the key challenges in recent conflicts has been the high rate of multiple deployments, which can exacerbate mental health issues. Service members returning from combat zones often face difficulties readjusting to civilian life, and the cumulative stress of repeated deployments can take a significant toll on mental health.

The mental health issues faced by veterans of the Gulf War, Iraq, and Afghanistan include not only PTSD but also other conditions such as depression, anxiety, and substance use disorders. The physical injuries sustained in combat, including TBI, have further complicated the mental health landscape for these veterans.

Advances in Diagnosis, Treatment, and Policy Changes

Advancements in diagnosis and treatment have significantly improved outcomes for those affected by combat-related mental health issues. Evidence-based therapies such as Cognitive Behavioral Therapy (CBT) and Eye Movement Desensitization and Reprocessing (EMDR) have been effective in treating PTSD. Additionally, pharmacological treatments have been refined to better manage symptoms of depression and anxiety.

Policy changes have also played a crucial role in improving mental health care for military personnel and veterans. Initiatives such as the Mental

Health Parity Act and the establishment of comprehensive VA mental health programs have increased access to care and support for those in need.

The VA has developed specialized programs for addressing the unique needs of veterans, including those with PTSD and TBI. These programs focus on early identification and intervention, providing comprehensive care that includes mental health services, rehabilitation, and support for reintegration into civilian life.

Recent years have also seen an increased emphasis on the importance of mental health education and training within the military. Efforts to destigmatize mental health issues and promote help-seeking behaviors are critical to ensuring that service members receive the care they need.

The establishment of the VA's National Center for PTSD has been a significant development in the field. The center conducts research, provides education, and develops treatment guidelines to improve the care of veterans with PTSD. Its work has helped to advance the understanding of trauma-related mental health issues and promote best practices in treatment.

Impact of Military Culture on Mental Health:

Military Culture and Stigma

Military culture has a significant impact on the mental health of service members. The emphasis on strength, resilience, and self-reliance can create barriers to seeking help for mental health issues. Stigma surrounding mental illness remains a challenge, with many service members fearing that acknowledging their struggles could harm their careers.

The military's focus on mission readiness and operational effectiveness often means that mental health issues are viewed as potential liabilities. Service members may be reluctant to seek help due to concerns about being perceived as weak or unfit for duty. This stigma can prevent individuals from accessing the support and treatment they need.

Efforts to change cultural perceptions within the military are ongoing. Programs aimed at reducing stigma and promoting mental health awareness are critical to encouraging service members to seek help. Leaders within the military are increasingly recognizing the importance of mental health and advocating for supportive environments.

The military's emphasis on discipline, toughness, and perseverance can create an environment where mental health struggles are seen as signs of weakness. This perception is reinforced by concerns about career advancement and the potential impact of mental health diagnoses on security clearances and deployability.

The stigma surrounding mental health issues can also extend to families and communities, further isolating service members who may be struggling. Addressing this stigma requires a comprehensive approach that includes education, support, and leadership engagement.

Efforts to Change Cultural Perceptions and Improve Mental Health Care

Numerous initiatives have been implemented to improve mental health care and change cultural perceptions within the military. These efforts include training programs for leaders, mental health awareness campaigns, and the integration of mental health professionals within military units.

The focus on building a culture of support and understanding is essential for ensuring that service members receive the care they need. By addressing stigma and promoting mental health as a critical component of overall readiness, the military can better support the well-being of its personnel.

Programs such as the Comprehensive Soldier and Family Fitness program (CSF2) and the Real Warriors Campaign have been instrumental in promoting mental health awareness and resilience within the military community. These initiatives emphasize the importance of seeking help and provide resources to support mental health and well-being.

The integration of mental health professionals within military units has also been a key strategy for improving access to care. Embedded mental health providers can offer timely and confidential support, helping to address issues before they escalate. This approach ensures that mental health care is readily available and integrated into the daily lives of service members.

Efforts to change cultural perceptions within the military also include initiatives to promote leadership engagement and support. Leaders play a crucial role in shaping the culture of their units and encouraging help-seeking behaviors. Training programs for leaders emphasize the importance of mental health awareness, reducing stigma, and creating a supportive environment for service members.

The historical overview of military and veteran mental health highlights the significant progress made in understanding and addressing the unique mental health needs of service members. From the early days of limited recognition and harsh treatments to the modern era of comprehensive care and support, the journey reflects broader changes in societal attitudes and medical knowledge.

While significant advancements have been made, ongoing efforts are needed to ensure that mental health care is accessible, effective, and free from stigma. The following chapters will delve deeper into the current mental health crisis among military veterans, exploring the challenges and solutions in greater detail.

The history of military and veteran mental health care underscores the importance of continued advocacy, research, and innovation. By building on the progress made and addressing the challenges that remain, we can work towards a future where all service members and veterans receive the mental health care and support they deserve.

Chapter 4

The Stigma of Men Discussing Their Feelings

Introduction to Stigma

Stigma is a powerful social force that can significantly impact individuals' lives, especially when it comes to mental health. For men, discussing feelings and mental health issues often carries a particular stigma rooted in traditional notions of masculinity and strength. This chapter explores the cultural and social roots of this stigma, its impact on mental health, and the efforts to break the silence and change perspectives. By understanding the origins and effects of stigma, we can work towards creating a more supportive environment for men to openly discuss their mental health.

Stigma surrounding mental health can take many forms, including societal attitudes, self-stigma, and structural barriers. For men, these forms of stigma are often intertwined with expectations about gender roles and behaviors. Understanding how stigma operates and its impact on men's mental health is crucial for addressing the mental health crisis and promoting well-being.

Cultural and Social Roots of Stigma:

Historical Perspectives on Masculinity and Emotional Expression

The roots of stigma against men discussing their feelings can be traced back to historical perspectives on masculinity. Traditional views of masculinity often emphasize traits such as stoicism, emotional restraint, and self-reliance. These traits have been idealized in many cultures, creating an expectation that men should be strong, unemotional, and independent.

Throughout history, expressions of vulnerability and emotional openness have been associated with femininity, while traits like toughness and emotional control have been linked to masculinity. This dichotomy has contributed to a cultural norm where men feel pressured to suppress their emotions and avoid seeking help for mental health issues.

In many cultures, the ideal of the "strong, silent type" has been perpetuated through literature, art, and social norms. Historical figures and fictional heroes who embody this ideal have reinforced the notion that real men do not show weakness or express emotional pain. This cultural narrative has had a lasting impact on how men perceive and respond to their own mental health needs.

Historical events and movements have also influenced perceptions of masculinity. For instance, the Industrial Revolution emphasized physical labor and self-sufficiency, further entrenching the idea that men should be strong and resilient. Similarly, wartime experiences and the portrayal of soldiers as stoic and unflinching in the face of adversity reinforced these norms.

Societal Expectations and Norms Regarding Male Behavior

Societal expectations and norms play a significant role in reinforcing stigma. From a young age, boys are often socialized to conform to traditional gender roles that discourage emotional expression. Phrases like "boys don't cry" and "man up" are commonly used to reinforce the idea that expressing emotions is a sign of weakness.

These societal messages can have profound effects on boys and men, leading them to internalize the belief that they must handle their problems alone and avoid appearing vulnerable. This internalized stigma can prevent men from seeking help for mental health issues, as they may fear judgment, ridicule, or rejection.

The pressure to conform to societal expectations can also lead to unhealthy coping mechanisms, such as substance abuse, aggression, or social withdrawal. These behaviors can further exacerbate mental health problems and create a cycle of stigma and suffering.

The workplace and other social environments often reinforce these norms. In many professional settings, showing vulnerability or discussing mental health issues can be perceived as unprofessional or a sign of weakness. This perception can discourage men from seeking support or disclosing their struggles, further perpetuating the stigma.

Educational institutions also play a role in perpetuating these norms. Boys and young men are often encouraged to excel in sports and academics while being discouraged from expressing emotions or seeking help for mental health issues. This can lead to the development of harmful coping mechanisms and a reluctance to seek help later in life.

The Role of Media and Popular Culture in Reinforcing Stigma

Media and popular culture play a crucial role in shaping societal attitudes towards mental health and masculinity. Television shows, movies, and advertisements often depict men as stoic, self-reliant, and emotionally detached. These portrayals reinforce the stereotype that men should not express their emotions or seek help for mental health issues.

Popular culture often glorifies male characters who embody traditional masculine traits while portraying emotionally expressive men as weak or flawed. This representation can create unrealistic and harmful expectations for men, making it difficult for them to navigate their emotional lives authentically.

However, media and popular culture also have the potential to challenge these stereotypes and promote healthier attitudes towards men's mental health. In recent years, there has been a growing movement to depict more diverse and nuanced representations of masculinity. Films, television shows, and advertisements that showcase men expressing vulnerability and seeking help can play a powerful role in reducing stigma.

By highlighting positive examples of men discussing their feelings and addressing mental health issues, media can contribute to changing societal attitudes and encouraging more open conversations about mental health.

For example, recent films like "A Beautiful Mind" and "Good Will Hunting" have portrayed male characters struggling with mental health issues and seeking help. These portrayals can help normalize mental health struggles and encourage men to seek support.

Social media platforms also play a significant role in shaping attitudes towards mental health. While social media can perpetuate stigma, it also provides opportunities for raising awareness and promoting mental health initiatives. Influencers and public figures who openly discuss their mental health struggles can help challenge stigma and encourage their followers to seek help.

Impact of Stigma on Mental Health:

Psychological and Emotional Consequences of Stigma

The stigma surrounding men's mental health can have severe psychological and emotional consequences. Men who feel pressured to conform to traditional masculine norms may suppress their emotions and avoid seeking help, leading to increased feelings of isolation, anxiety, and depression.

The internalization of stigma can result in self-stigma, where men view their mental health struggles as personal failures or weaknesses. This self-stigma can exacerbate mental health issues, creating a cycle of shame and silence that is difficult to break.

Studies have shown that men who adhere strongly to traditional masculine norms are less likely to seek help for mental health issues and are at greater risk for negative mental health outcomes. The pressure to appear strong and self-reliant can prevent men from accessing the support they need, leading to a worsening of symptoms and a decreased quality of life.

The emotional toll of stigma can also manifest in physical symptoms. Chronic stress, anxiety, and depression can lead to physical health problems, such as cardiovascular disease, weakened immune function, and chronic pain. The interplay between mental and physical health highlights the importance of addressing stigma and promoting mental well-being.

Men who suppress their emotions may also experience difficulty in forming and maintaining healthy relationships. The inability to express vulnerability and seek support can lead to relationship conflicts, further exacerbating feelings of isolation and distress.

Barriers to Seeking Help and Treatment

Stigma creates significant barriers to seeking help and treatment for mental health issues. Men who fear judgment or ridicule may avoid disclosing their struggles to friends, family, or healthcare providers. This reluctance to seek help can result in untreated mental health conditions and a decline in overall well-being.

Barriers to seeking help are compounded by structural factors, such as a lack of accessible mental health services and inadequate support systems. In many cases, men may not know where to turn for help or may face long wait times and high costs for mental health care. These barriers can further discourage men from seeking the support they need.

The fear of being perceived as weak or unfit can also deter men from seeking help within professional environments, including the military and workplace settings. Concerns about career advancement, job security, and social standing can prevent men from accessing mental health services and disclosing their struggles.

The stigma surrounding mental health can also impact the quality of care that men receive. Healthcare providers may hold biases or assumptions about men and mental health, leading to misdiagnosis or inadequate treatment. Addressing these biases and promoting gender-sensitive approaches to mental health care are essential for improving outcomes.

Workplace cultures that prioritize productivity and resilience over well-being can further perpetuate stigma. Men may feel pressured to hide their mental health struggles to avoid being perceived as less competent or capable. This can lead to burnout, decreased job satisfaction, and reduced productivity.

Case Studies and Statistics on the Impact of Stigma

Research and case studies highlight the profound impact of stigma on men's mental health. Studies have shown that men are less likely than women to seek help for mental health issues, and when they do seek help, they often wait until their symptoms are severe.

For example, a study conducted by the National Institute of Mental Health found that men are less likely than women to receive treatment for depression, even though they may experience similar levels of distress. This disparity in treatment-seeking behavior is largely attributed to stigma and traditional gender norms.

Case studies of men who have overcome stigma and sought help for their mental health provide valuable insights into the challenges and triumphs of addressing stigma. These stories highlight the importance of support, education, and advocacy in encouraging men to seek help and break the cycle of silence.

Statistics on suicide rates among men further underscore the impact of stigma. Men are more likely than women to die by suicide, a trend that is partly attributed to the reluctance to seek help and the use of more lethal means. Addressing stigma and promoting mental health support are critical for reducing suicide rates and saving lives.

For instance, the Centers for Disease Control and Prevention (CDC) reports that men are nearly four times more likely than women to die by suicide. This alarming statistic underscores the need for targeted interventions to address the stigma and barriers that prevent men from seeking help.

Case studies of men who have successfully navigated their mental health challenges and sought support can serve as powerful examples for others. These stories can help normalize the experience of seeking help and provide hope and encouragement to those who may be struggling in silence.

Breaking the Silence: Changing Perspectives:

Efforts to Challenge and Reduce Stigma

Efforts to challenge and reduce stigma surrounding men's mental health are crucial for fostering a more supportive and open environment. Advocacy groups, public awareness campaigns, and mental health organizations play a vital role in changing societal attitudes and promoting mental well-being.

Campaigns such as Movember and Time to Change have been instrumental in raising awareness about men's mental health and encouraging open conversations. These initiatives use a variety of strategies, including social media campaigns, public events, and educational materials, to challenge stigma and promote help-seeking behaviors.

Mental health organizations also work to provide resources and support for men experiencing mental health issues. Programs that offer peer support, counseling, and educational workshops can help men feel more comfortable discussing their mental health and accessing the care they need.

The role of influential figures, such as athletes, celebrities, and public leaders, in challenging stigma cannot be overstated. When well-known individuals openly discuss their mental health struggles and advocate for mental well-being, they help to normalize these conversations and reduce stigma for others.

Public awareness campaigns that feature personal stories of men who have overcome mental health challenges can be particularly impactful. These stories can help break down barriers and encourage others to seek help by showing that they are not alone and that recovery is possible.

Role of Advocacy Groups and Public Awareness Campaigns

Advocacy groups and public awareness campaigns are at the forefront of efforts to reduce stigma and promote mental health. These organizations work to change societal attitudes, provide support and resources, and advocate for policy changes that improve access to mental health care.

Organizations like the National Alliance on Mental Illness (NAMI) and Mental Health America (MHA) offer a range of programs and initiatives aimed at reducing stigma and supporting individuals with mental health issues. These organizations provide educational materials, support groups, and advocacy resources to help individuals and communities address mental health stigma.

Public awareness campaigns use various strategies to reach diverse audiences and promote mental health awareness. Social media campaigns, public service announcements, and community events are effective tools for raising awareness and encouraging open conversations about mental health.

The impact of these campaigns is evident in the growing public awareness and acceptance of mental health issues. As more people become informed about mental health and the importance of seeking help, the stigma surrounding these issues begins to diminish, creating a more supportive environment for those in need.

For example, the "It's Okay to Talk" campaign by the Campaign Against Living Miserably (CALM) uses social media and public events to encourage men to open up about their mental health. By normalizing these conversations and providing resources, the campaign aims to reduce stigma and promote help-seeking behaviors.

Impact of Social Movements and Changing Cultural Norms

Social movements and changing cultural norms have played a significant role in reducing stigma and promoting mental health awareness. Movements such as MeToo and Black Lives Matter have brought attention to the intersection of mental health with issues of gender, race, and social justice, highlighting the importance of addressing mental health within broader societal contexts.

The growing emphasis on mental health as a critical component of overall well-being reflects a shift in cultural norms. Increasingly, mental health is being recognized as essential to a healthy and fulfilling life, and discussions about mental health are becoming more common and accepted.

This cultural shift is evident in the increasing number of workplaces, schools, and community organizations that prioritize mental health. Initiatives that promote mental health education, provide resources, and support open conversations are becoming more prevalent, contributing to a more inclusive and supportive environment.

As cultural norms continue to evolve, the stigma surrounding men's mental health is gradually diminishing. By promoting open dialogue, challenging harmful stereotypes, and advocating for mental health awareness, social movements and cultural changes are helping to create a more supportive and inclusive society.

The influence of social movements can also be seen in policy changes and legislative efforts to improve mental health care. Advocacy for mental health parity, improved access to care, and support for marginalized communities are all part of the broader effort to reduce stigma and promote mental well-being.

Strategies for Fostering Open Conversations:

Creating Supportive Environments for Men to Discuss Mental Health

Creating supportive environments for men to discuss their mental health is essential for reducing stigma and promoting well-being. Supportive environments include safe spaces where men feel comfortable sharing their experiences, receiving validation, and accessing resources.

Support groups, both in-person and online, provide valuable opportunities for men to connect with others who share similar experiences. These groups offer a sense of community and support, helping men feel less isolated and more understood. Peer support programs, where individuals with lived experience provide guidance and encouragement, can also be highly effective.

Workplaces, schools, and community organizations play a crucial role in creating supportive environments. By promoting mental health awareness, offering resources, and fostering open conversations, these institutions can help reduce stigma and encourage help-seeking behaviors.

Family and friends also play a critical role in creating supportive environments. By offering understanding, empathy, and encouragement, loved ones can help men feel more comfortable discussing their mental health and seeking support.

In addition to support groups, mentorship programs can provide valuable guidance and support for men navigating mental health challenges. Mentors who have experienced similar struggles can offer insights, encouragement, and practical advice, helping mentees feel more empowered to seek help and take steps towards recovery.

Role of Education and Mental Health Literacy

Education and mental health literacy are key components of efforts to reduce stigma and promote open conversations about mental health. Providing accurate information about mental health, challenging myths and misconceptions, and promoting help-seeking behaviors are essential for fostering a supportive environment.

Educational programs that focus on mental health awareness can be implemented in schools, workplaces, and community organizations. These programs should aim to increase understanding of mental health issues, reduce stigma, and provide information about available resources and support.

Mental health literacy campaigns can use various media, including social media, websites, and printed materials, to reach diverse audiences. By providing accessible and accurate information, these campaigns can help individuals recognize the signs of mental health issues and understand the importance of seeking help.

Training programs for healthcare providers, educators, and community leaders are also essential for promoting mental health literacy. These programs should emphasize the importance of a compassionate and non-judgmental approach to mental health, helping to create a more supportive environment for individuals seeking care.

Educational initiatives that involve storytelling and personal narratives can be particularly effective in promoting mental health literacy. Hearing real-life stories of individuals who have navigated mental health challenges and found support can help break down stigma and inspire others to seek help.

Practical Tips for Encouraging Open Dialogue

Encouraging open dialogue about mental health requires a proactive approach and the implementation of practical strategies. Here are some tips for fostering open conversations about mental health:

1. **Normalize Mental Health Conversations:** Treat discussions about mental health as a normal and important part of overall well-being. By incorporating mental health into everyday conversations, you can help reduce stigma and create a more open environment.

2. **Use Inclusive Language:** Use language that is inclusive and non-judgmental when discussing mental health. Avoid terms that reinforce stigma or negative stereotypes, and instead use language that promotes understanding and empathy.

3. **Share Personal Stories:** Sharing personal experiences with mental health can help break down barriers and encourage others to open up. Personal stories provide powerful examples of resilience and recovery, helping to reduce stigma and promote help-seeking behaviors.

4. **Provide Resources and Support:** Offer information about available mental health resources and support services. Providing practical assistance, such as contact information for mental health professionals or support groups, can help individuals access the care they need.

5. **Create Safe Spaces:** Establish safe and confidential spaces where individuals can discuss their mental health without fear of judgment or repercussion. This can include support groups, counseling services, or designated areas in workplaces and schools.

6. **Encourage Active Listening:** Practice active listening by giving your full attention, showing empathy, and validating the experiences of others. Active listening helps build trust and creates a supportive environment for open conversations.

7. **Promote Mental Health Education:** Advocate for mental health education and training programs in your community. Increasing mental health literacy can help reduce stigma and promote a more supportive environment for discussing mental health.

8. **Lead by Example:** Model healthy behaviors and attitudes towards mental health by being open about your own experiences and

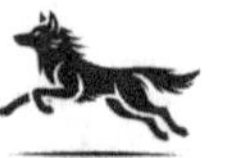

encouraging others to do the same. Leading by example can inspire others to speak up and seek support.

By implementing these strategies and fostering a culture of openness and support, we can help reduce the stigma surrounding men's mental health and promote well-being for all individuals.

Encouraging open dialogue also involves recognizing and addressing the unique challenges faced by different groups of men, including men of color, LGBTQ+ men, and men from various cultural backgrounds. Tailoring approaches to meet the specific needs of these groups is essential for creating inclusive and effective support systems.

The stigma surrounding men's mental health is deeply rooted in cultural and social norms that emphasize traditional notions of masculinity and strength. This stigma can have profound psychological and emotional consequences, creating barriers to seeking help and treatment. However, efforts to challenge and reduce stigma are making a significant impact, promoting open conversations and creating supportive environments for men to discuss their mental health.

By understanding the roots and impact of stigma, and by implementing strategies to foster open dialogue, we can work towards a future where men feel comfortable and supported in discussing their mental health. The next chapter will delve into the current mental health crisis among men in the USA, exploring the specific challenges and solutions in greater detail.

Creating a society where men can freely discuss their mental health and seek support requires ongoing effort and collaboration. By continuing to challenge stigma, promote mental health literacy, and create supportive environments, we can help ensure that all individuals have the opportunity to achieve mental well-being and lead fulfilling lives.

Chapter 5

Current Mental Health Crisis Among Men in the USA

Introduction to the Current Mental Health Crisis

The mental health crisis among men in the United States has reached alarming levels, with significant implications for individuals, families, communities, and society as a whole. Despite increasing awareness and advances in treatment, many men continue to struggle with mental health issues in silence, often due to stigma and barriers to accessing care. This chapter explores the prevalence of mental health disorders among men, the factors contributing to these issues, and the broader societal impact.

Men's mental health is a critical public health concern that demands urgent attention. Addressing the mental health crisis among men is not only essential for improving individual well-being but also for enhancing the overall health and productivity of society. By examining the current landscape and identifying key challenges, we can develop targeted interventions to support men's mental health.

Prevalence of Mental Health Issues Among Men

Statistics on Depression, Anxiety, and Other Mental Health Disorders

Mental health disorders are prevalent among men in the United States, with depression and anxiety being among the most common conditions. According to the National Institute of Mental Health (NIMH), approximately 6 million men in the U.S. experience depression each year, and more than 3 million suffer from anxiety disorders.

Depression in men often presents differently than in women, with symptoms such as irritability, anger, and aggression being more common. Men are also more likely to report physical symptoms such as headaches, digestive issues, and chronic pain. These differences in symptom presentation can lead to underdiagnosis and undertreatment of depression in men.

Anxiety disorders, including generalized anxiety disorder, panic disorder, and social anxiety disorder, are also significant concerns for men. These conditions can severely impact daily functioning, relationships, and overall quality of life. Despite the prevalence of anxiety disorders, many men do not seek treatment, often due to stigma and a reluctance to appear vulnerable.

In addition to depression and anxiety, men are at risk for other mental health disorders, such as bipolar disorder, post-traumatic stress disorder (PTSD), and substance use disorders. These conditions can have devastating effects on men's lives and require comprehensive and accessible mental health care.

Substance use disorders, including alcohol and drug addiction, are particularly prevalent among men. The Substance Abuse and Mental Health Services Administration (SAMHSA) reports that men are more likely than women to use nearly all types of illicit drugs and are more likely to need emergency department visits for overdose. Substance use disorders often co-occur with other mental health conditions, exacerbating the overall mental health crisis among men.

Analysis of Suicide Rates and Contributing Factors

One of the most alarming aspects of the mental health crisis among men is the high rate of suicide. According to the Centers for Disease Control and Prevention (CDC), men are nearly four times more likely than women to die by suicide. In 2019, men accounted for 79% of all suicide deaths in the United States, with the highest rates among middle-aged white men.

Several factors contribute to the high suicide rates among men, including untreated mental health conditions, substance abuse, social isolation, and access to lethal means. Men are more likely to use firearms in suicide attempts, which increases the likelihood of a fatal outcome. The reluctance to seek help and the stigma surrounding mental health issues further exacerbate the risk of suicide.

Understanding the contributing factors to suicide among men is essential for developing effective prevention strategies. These strategies must address the unique challenges men face, including the stigma of seeking help, the cultural pressures to appear strong, and the need for accessible and targeted mental health services.

The role of economic factors in suicide rates among men cannot be overlooked. Financial stress, unemployment, and job insecurity are significant risk factors for suicide. Economic downturns and periods of financial instability have been linked to increased suicide rates, highlighting the importance of addressing economic stressors as part of suicide prevention efforts.

The COVID-19 pandemic has also had a significant impact on suicide rates among men. The pandemic has exacerbated feelings of isolation, anxiety, and hopelessness, contributing to an increase in mental health issues and suicide risk. The pandemic's economic impact, including job loss and financial hardship, has further heightened the risk of suicide among men.

Factors Contributing to Mental Health Issues:

Socioeconomic Factors (Unemployment, Financial Stress)

Socioeconomic factors play a significant role in men's mental health. Unemployment, financial stress, and job insecurity are major contributors to mental health issues. Men who are unemployed or facing financial difficulties are at a higher risk for depression, anxiety, and substance use disorders.

The loss of a job can lead to a loss of identity and purpose, particularly for men who derive a sense of self-worth from their careers. Financial stress can also strain relationships and contribute to feelings of hopelessness and despair. The economic uncertainty created by the COVID-19 pandemic has further exacerbated these issues, with many men experiencing job loss and financial hardship.

Addressing the mental health impact of socioeconomic factors requires comprehensive strategies that include economic support, job training, and mental health services. Providing resources and support to men facing financial stress can help mitigate the negative impact on mental health and promote resilience.

Programs that offer financial counseling, employment assistance, and support for career transitions can be valuable resources for men facing economic challenges. Additionally, policies that promote job security, fair wages, and access to affordable healthcare are essential for supporting men's mental health and well-being.

Cultural and Societal Pressures

Cultural and societal pressures to conform to traditional masculine norms can have a profound impact on men's mental health. The expectation to be strong, self-reliant, and unemotional can prevent men from seeking help and expressing their feelings. These pressures can lead to internalized stigma and self-criticism, contributing to mental health issues.

The concept of "toxic masculinity" refers to cultural norms that encourage harmful behaviors and attitudes, such as aggression, suppression of emotions, and dominance. These norms can negatively impact men's mental health and relationships, leading to increased stress, isolation, and conflict.

Challenging and changing cultural and societal norms requires a multi-faceted approach that includes education, advocacy, and the promotion of positive models of masculinity. Encouraging men to embrace a broader range of emotional expression and seeking help can contribute to better mental health outcomes.

The impact of media and popular culture on men's mental health cannot be overlooked. Media portrayals of men as stoic, invulnerable, and self-sufficient reinforce harmful stereotypes and discourage men from seeking help. Efforts to promote diverse and positive representations of masculinity in the media can help challenge these stereotypes and support men's mental health.

Racial and Ethnic Disparities

Racial and ethnic disparities in mental health care access and outcomes are significant concerns. Men of color, including African American, Hispanic, Asian, and Native American men, face unique challenges that impact their mental health. These challenges include discrimination, systemic racism, and cultural barriers to seeking help.

African American men, for example, are less likely to seek mental health treatment and are more likely to experience severe symptoms of mental health disorders. Cultural stigma, mistrust of the healthcare system, and a lack of culturally competent providers contribute to these disparities.

Addressing racial and ethnic disparities in mental health requires targeted interventions that consider the cultural context and specific needs of different communities. Increasing the availability of culturally competent mental health services and promoting mental health awareness within communities of color are essential steps.

Community-based mental health initiatives that involve collaboration with local organizations, faith-based groups, and cultural leaders can be effective in addressing the unique mental health needs of men of color. These initiatives can help build trust, reduce stigma, and provide culturally relevant support and resources.

Impact of the COVID-19 Pandemic

The COVID-19 pandemic has had a profound impact on mental health worldwide, with men in the United States being no exception. The pandemic has exacerbated existing mental health issues and created new challenges, such as social isolation, financial stress, and health-related anxiety.

Men have faced unique challenges during the pandemic, including increased rates of unemployment and financial hardship, disruptions to daily routines, and the added stress of managing family responsibilities. The uncertainty and fear associated with the pandemic have also contributed to increased levels of anxiety and depression.

The pandemic has highlighted the importance of accessible mental health care and the need for flexible and innovative approaches to support mental well-being. Telehealth services, virtual support groups, and online mental health resources have become essential tools for providing care and support during these challenging times.

The long-term impact of the COVID-19 pandemic on men's mental health is still unfolding. Continued efforts to provide mental health support, address economic challenges, and promote resilience are essential for mitigating the pandemic's impact on mental health.

Societal Impact of Men's Mental Health Crisis:

Economic Costs of Untreated Mental Health Issues

Untreated mental health issues among men have significant economic costs. These costs include lost productivity, increased healthcare expenses, and the financial burden on families and communities. The economic impact of mental health issues underscores the importance of investing in mental health care and prevention.

Men with untreated mental health conditions may struggle to maintain employment, leading to decreased productivity and increased absenteeism.

The inability to work can result in financial instability and increased reliance on social services. The cost of untreated mental health issues also extends to healthcare, as individuals with mental health conditions are more likely to experience physical health problems and require medical care.

Investing in mental health care and early intervention can reduce these economic costs and improve overall well-being. Programs that provide mental health support in the workplace, access to affordable mental health services, and prevention initiatives can contribute to a healthier and more productive society.

Employers can play a significant role in addressing the economic costs of mental health issues by implementing workplace mental health programs. These programs can include employee assistance programs (EAPs), mental health training for managers, and initiatives to promote work-life balance and stress management.

Effects on Families and Communities

The mental health crisis among men has far-reaching effects on families and communities. Men who struggle with mental health issues may experience difficulties in their relationships, impacting their partners, children, and extended family members. The strain on relationships can lead to increased conflict, emotional distress, and disruptions in family functioning.

Children of men with untreated mental health conditions may also be affected, experiencing emotional and behavioral challenges. The intergenerational impact of mental health issues highlights the importance of providing support and resources to families to promote overall well-being.

Communities also bear the burden of untreated mental health issues, with increased rates of substance abuse, violence, and homelessness. The societal impact of men's mental health underscores the need for community-based interventions and support systems to address these challenges.

Community mental health initiatives that involve collaboration between mental health professionals, community organizations, and local government can be effective in addressing the broader impact of men's mental health issues. These initiatives can provide support, education, and resources to individuals and families, helping to build resilient communities.

Workplace Implications

Mental health issues among men have significant implications for the workplace. Employees struggling with mental health conditions may experience decreased productivity, increased absenteeism, and difficulties in maintaining job performance. The stigma surrounding mental health can also prevent men from seeking help, leading to further challenges in the workplace.

Employers play a crucial role in supporting men's mental health by creating a supportive and inclusive work environment. This includes providing access to mental health resources, promoting work-life balance, and fostering a culture of openness and support. Workplace mental health programs and employee assistance programs (EAPs) can provide valuable support and resources for employees.

Addressing mental health in the workplace benefits both employees and employers by promoting well-being, reducing absenteeism, and enhancing productivity. Employers who prioritize mental health create a positive and supportive work environment that benefits the entire organization.

Workplace policies that promote mental health awareness, provide flexible work arrangements, and support employees in managing stress and work-life balance are essential for creating a mentally healthy workplace. Training managers to recognize and respond to mental health issues can also help create a supportive and inclusive work environment.

Barriers to Accessing Mental Health Care:

Financial and Insurance Barriers

Financial and insurance barriers are significant obstacles to accessing mental health care for many men. The cost of mental health services, including therapy and medication, can be prohibitive for individuals without adequate insurance coverage. High out-of-pocket costs and limited coverage for mental health services can prevent men from seeking the care they need.

Insurance barriers, such as limited provider networks and restrictions on the number of covered sessions, can also hinder access to mental health care. Men with high-deductible health plans or no insurance may delay or forgo treatment due to financial constraints.

Addressing financial and insurance barriers requires policy changes and initiatives to increase access to affordable mental health care. Expanding insurance coverage for mental health services, providing financial assistance programs, and advocating for mental health parity are essential steps to ensure that all individuals can access the care they need.

The implementation of the Mental Health Parity and Addiction Equity Act (MHPAEA) has been a significant step towards addressing insurance barriers by requiring that mental health and substance use disorder benefits be no more restrictive than medical/surgical benefits. Continued efforts to enforce and expand parity laws are essential for improving access to mental health care.

Availability of Mental Health Services

The availability of mental health services is another critical barrier to accessing care. In many areas, particularly rural and underserved communities, there is a shortage of mental health providers. Long wait times for appointments and limited availability of specialized services can prevent men from receiving timely and appropriate care.

The lack of culturally competent providers can also impact access to mental health services for men from diverse backgrounds. Men who do not see providers who understand their cultural context and specific needs may be less likely to seek and continue treatment.

Increasing the availability of mental health services requires investment in the mental health workforce, including training and recruitment of providers. Expanding telehealth services and integrating mental health care into primary care settings can also help address gaps in service availability.

Telehealth has become an increasingly important tool for expanding access to mental health care, particularly during the COVID-19 pandemic. Telehealth services can provide convenient and accessible care, reducing barriers related to transportation, scheduling, and geographic location.

Stigma and Self-Stigma

Stigma and self-stigma remain significant barriers to accessing mental health care for men. The fear of being judged or perceived as weak can prevent men from seeking help and disclosing their mental health struggles. Self-stigma, where individuals internalize negative attitudes about mental health, can also hinder help-seeking behaviors.

Addressing stigma requires comprehensive strategies that include public awareness campaigns, education, and advocacy. Promoting positive models of masculinity and encouraging open conversations about mental health can help reduce stigma and support help-seeking behaviors.

Efforts to reduce stigma should also focus on creating supportive environments where men feel comfortable discussing their mental health. This includes fostering a culture of acceptance and understanding in workplaces, schools, and communities.

Programs that involve peer support and mentorship can be particularly effective in addressing stigma. Men who have successfully navigated mental health challenges and are willing to share their experiences can serve as role models and provide valuable support to others facing similar struggles.

Specific Challenges for Men of Color and LGBTQ+ Men

Men of color and LGBTQ+ men face specific challenges in accessing mental health care. These challenges include discrimination, cultural stigma, and a lack of culturally competent providers. Addressing these unique barriers requires targeted interventions and culturally sensitive approaches.

Men of color may experience additional barriers to accessing mental health care due to systemic racism and historical mistrust of the healthcare system. Providing culturally competent care and building trust within communities of color are essential steps to improve access and outcomes.

LGBTQ+ men face unique mental health challenges, including higher rates of depression, anxiety, and suicide. Discrimination, social stigma, and a lack of inclusive mental health services can prevent LGBTQ+ men from seeking help. Providing affirming and inclusive care is critical for supporting the mental health of LGBTQ+ men.

Programs that provide targeted support and resources for men of color and LGBTQ+ men can help address these specific challenges. Community-based initiatives, peer support programs, and advocacy efforts are essential for promoting mental health and well-being for all individuals.

Collaborations between mental health organizations, community leaders, and advocacy groups can help ensure that mental health services are accessible and responsive to the needs of diverse populations. Training providers in cultural competency and inclusive care practices is also essential for improving the quality of mental health care for all individuals.

The current mental health crisis among men in the United States is a complex and multifaceted issue that requires urgent attention. The prevalence of mental health disorders, high suicide rates, and significant barriers to accessing care highlight the need for comprehensive and targeted interventions. By addressing the unique challenges men face and promoting mental health awareness, we can work towards a future where all men have access to the support and care they need.

The next chapter will delve into the suicide rates among men in the USA, exploring the factors contributing to this crisis and the strategies for prevention and support. Addressing the mental health needs of men is essential for promoting well-being and building a healthier and more resilient society.

Creating a society where men can freely discuss their mental health and seek support requires ongoing effort and collaboration. By continuing to challenge stigma, promote mental health literacy, and create supportive environments, we can help ensure that all individuals have the opportunity to achieve mental well-being and lead fulfilling lives.

Chapter 6

Suicide Rates Among Men in the USA

Introduction to Suicide Rates Among Men

Suicide is a major public health issue that has a profound impact on individuals, families, and communities. Among men in the United States, suicide rates are particularly high, representing a significant portion of the overall suicide deaths. This chapter explores the statistical trends, contributing factors, and prevention strategies related to suicide among men.

The high rate of suicide among men is a critical concern that demands urgent attention. Understanding the factors that contribute to this crisis and implementing effective prevention strategies are essential steps toward reducing suicide rates and promoting mental health and well-being.

Statistical Trends and Demographic Analysis:

Breakdown of Suicide Rates by Age, Race, and Geographic Location

Suicide rates among men vary significantly by age, race, and geographic location. According to the Centers for Disease Control and Prevention (CDC), men accounted for nearly 80% of all suicide deaths in the United States in 2019. The highest suicide rates are observed among middle-aged and older men, particularly those aged 45-64 and 85 and older.

In terms of racial and ethnic disparities, white men have the highest suicide rates, followed by Native American, African American, Hispanic, and Asian men. Cultural factors, socioeconomic status, and access to mental health services contribute to these disparities.

Geographic location also plays a role in suicide rates, with higher rates observed in rural areas compared to urban areas. Factors such as social isolation, limited access to healthcare, and economic stressors contribute to the elevated suicide risk in rural communities.

The CDC's data indicates that suicide rates have been increasing over the past two decades. This trend underscores the need for comprehensive and targeted interventions to address the factors contributing to high suicide rates among men.

Trends Over Time and Recent Changes

Over the past two decades, suicide rates among men have shown an upward trend, with significant increases observed in certain age groups and demographic categories. This increase is concerning and highlights the need for ongoing monitoring and research to understand the underlying causes and identify effective prevention strategies.

Recent changes in suicide rates have been influenced by various factors, including economic downturns, the opioid epidemic, and the COVID-19 pandemic. The economic challenges and social isolation brought about by these events have exacerbated mental health issues and increased the risk of suicide among men.

The COVID-19 pandemic has had a profound impact on mental health, with increased rates of anxiety, depression, and substance abuse reported. The pandemic's economic impact, including job loss and financial instability, has further heightened the risk of suicide among men. Addressing these challenges requires a multifaceted approach that includes economic support, mental health services, and public awareness campaigns.

Factors Contributing to High Suicide Rates:

Mental Health Disorders (Depression, Anxiety, PTSD)

Mental health disorders are a significant contributing factor to suicide among men. Depression, anxiety, and post-traumatic stress disorder (PTSD) are among the most common conditions associated with suicide risk. Men with these mental health disorders may experience feelings of hopelessness, worthlessness, and severe emotional pain, which can lead to suicidal thoughts and behaviors.

Depression is a leading risk factor for suicide, with studies showing that individuals with depression are significantly more likely to attempt suicide than those without the condition. Symptoms of depression in men, such as irritability, anger, and social withdrawal, can be particularly challenging to recognize and treat.

Anxiety disorders, including generalized anxiety disorder, panic disorder, and social anxiety disorder, also contribute to suicide risk. The intense fear, worry, and physical symptoms associated with anxiety disorders can lead to feelings of desperation and hopelessness.

PTSD, particularly among military veterans, is another critical factor contributing to suicide risk. The traumatic experiences associated with combat and military service can lead to severe and persistent mental health issues, including PTSD, which increases the risk of suicide.

Substance Abuse and Addiction

Substance abuse and addiction are closely linked to suicide risk among men. Alcohol and drug use can exacerbate mental health issues, impair judgment, and increase impulsivity, all of which contribute to the risk of suicide. Men are more likely than women to engage in substance use and to develop substance use disorders, which can have devastating effects on mental health.

The opioid epidemic has had a significant impact on suicide rates, with an increasing number of suicides involving opioid overdoses. The misuse of prescription medications, illicit drugs, and alcohol can lead to a cycle of addiction, mental health deterioration, and increased suicide risk.

Effective prevention and treatment of substance use disorders are essential components of suicide prevention strategies. Integrating mental health and substance use treatment services can help address the complex interplay between these issues and reduce the risk of suicide.

Social Isolation and Loneliness

Social isolation and loneliness are significant risk factors for suicide among men. Men who lack strong social connections and support networks are at a higher risk for mental health issues and suicidal behaviors. Social isolation can lead to feelings of loneliness, hopelessness, and despair, which can increase the risk of suicide.

The stigma surrounding mental health and the pressure to conform to traditional masculine norms can prevent men from seeking social support and forming meaningful connections. This isolation can be particularly pronounced in older men, who may experience loss of social connections due to retirement, bereavement, or health issues.

Addressing social isolation and loneliness requires initiatives that promote social connections, community engagement, and support networks. Programs that encourage men to participate in social activities, join support groups, and seek help can help reduce the risk of suicide.

Economic Stress and Unemployment

Economic stress and unemployment are major contributors to suicide risk among men. Financial difficulties, job loss, and job insecurity can lead to significant mental health challenges, including depression, anxiety, and suicidal thoughts. The loss of a job can also lead to a loss of identity, self-worth, and purpose, further exacerbating mental health issues.

Men who are unemployed or facing financial difficulties may experience increased stress, hopelessness, and despair. Economic stress can also strain relationships and contribute to feelings of isolation and loneliness.

The COVID-19 pandemic has further highlighted the impact of economic stress on mental health and suicide risk. The pandemic's economic impact, including widespread job loss and financial instability, has exacerbated mental health issues and increased the risk of suicide among men.

Addressing economic stress and unemployment as part of suicide prevention efforts requires comprehensive strategies that include economic support, job training, and mental health services. Providing resources and support to men facing financial stress can help mitigate the negative impact on mental health and reduce the risk of suicide.

Access to Lethal Means

Access to lethal means, such as firearms, is a significant risk factor for suicide among men. Men are more likely to use firearms in suicide attempts, which increases the likelihood of a fatal outcome. The availability and accessibility of firearms contribute to the high suicide rates among men.

Efforts to reduce access to lethal means, including safe storage practices and firearm safety education, are essential components of suicide prevention strategies. Implementing policies that promote responsible firearm ownership and reduce access to lethal means can help prevent suicide and save lives.

Public awareness campaigns that promote safe storage of firearms, as well

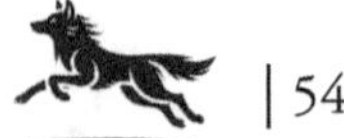

as initiatives that encourage individuals to seek help during times of crisis, can help reduce the risk of suicide. Collaborating with firearm owners, gun safety organizations, and mental health advocates can also support efforts to reduce access to lethal means and prevent suicide.

Suicide Among Military Veterans

Statistics on Veteran Suicide Rates

Military veterans are at a significantly higher risk for suicide compared to the general population. According to the Department of Veterans Affairs (VA), an average of 17 veterans die by suicide each day. The suicide rate among veterans is 1.5 times higher than that of non-veteran adults, with even higher rates observed among female veterans and younger veterans.

The unique challenges faced by veterans, including the transition to civilian life, combat-related trauma, and physical injuries, contribute to the elevated risk of suicide. The stigma surrounding mental health in the military and the barriers to accessing mental health care further exacerbate the risk of suicide among veterans.

Understanding the specific challenges and risk factors for veteran suicide is essential for developing targeted prevention strategies and providing the necessary support and resources to veterans in need.

Unique Challenges Faced by Veterans

Veterans face unique challenges that contribute to their elevated risk of suicide. These challenges include:

1. **Combat-Related Trauma:** Many veterans have experienced traumatic events during their military service, including combat, injury, and the loss of comrades. These experiences can lead to severe and persistent mental health issues, including PTSD, depression, and anxiety, which increase the risk of suicide.

2. **Transition to Civilian Life:** The transition from military to civilian life can be challenging for veterans. The loss of structure, purpose, and camaraderie can lead to feelings of isolation and identity loss. Veterans may also face difficulties finding employment, securing housing, and accessing healthcare, which can contribute to mental health issues and suicide risk.

3. **Physical Injuries and Chronic Pain:** Many veterans live with physical injuries and chronic pain resulting from their military service. These physical health issues can have a significant impact on mental health, leading to depression, anxiety, and increased suicide risk.

4. **Stigma and Barriers to Care:** The stigma surrounding mental health in the military and the barriers to accessing mental health care can prevent veterans from seeking help. Veterans may fear being perceived as weak or unfit for duty, leading to reluctance to disclose mental health struggles and seek treatment.

Addressing the unique challenges faced by veterans requires targeted interventions and support services that consider the specific needs and experiences of veterans. Providing comprehensive and accessible mental health care, promoting social connections, and supporting the transition to civilian life are essential steps in preventing veteran suicide.

Programs and Initiatives for Veteran Suicide Prevention

Several programs and initiatives have been developed to address the high suicide rates among veterans and provide support and resources to those in need. These programs include:

1. **Veterans Crisis Line:** The Veterans Crisis Line provides confidential support and crisis intervention services to veterans and their families. The hotline is available 24/7 and offers immediate assistance to veterans in crisis.

2. **VA Mental Health Services:** The VA provides a range of mental health services to veterans, including counseling, therapy, and medication management. The VA also offers specialized programs for veterans with PTSD, substance use disorders, and other mental health conditions.

3. **Community-Based Programs:** Community-based programs, such as Vet Centers and nonprofit organizations, provide support and resources to veterans. These programs offer counseling, peer support, and assistance with the transition to civilian life.

4. **Public Awareness Campaigns:** Public awareness campaigns, such as the "Be There" campaign, aim to raise awareness about veteran

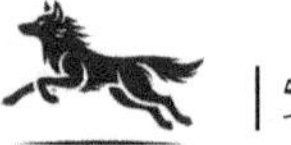

suicide and encourage individuals to support veterans in their communities. These campaigns promote the importance of social connections, mental health support, and seeking help.

5. **Collaborations with Military and Veteran Organizations:** Collaborations between military and veteran organizations, mental health providers, and policymakers are essential for addressing veteran suicide. These partnerships can help develop and implement effective prevention strategies, provide comprehensive support, and advocate for policy changes to improve access to care.

6. **MENtality Matters:** is a charity dedicated to supporting those men who are currently active US military personnel and Veterans alike. Through transformative retreats, engaging team-building events, and a thriving online community, MENtality Matters provides essential support and fosters a sense of camaraderie and brotherhood among those who have served. Their mission is to build better men by guiding them through 'The 4 Realms of Service: Personal, Relational, Professional, and Spiritual'. We believe that true growth and fulfillment come from a balanced development in these key areas. Through online coaching sessions, in-person team building events, and transformative retreats, we provide men with the tools and support they need to thrive in every aspect of their lives.

By providing targeted support and resources, promoting mental health awareness, and addressing the unique challenges faced by veterans, these programs and initiatives can help reduce the risk of suicide among veterans and support their overall well-being.

Prevention Strategies and Programs:

National and Community-Based Initiatives

National and community-based initiatives play a critical role in suicide prevention efforts. These initiatives aim to raise awareness, provide support and resources, and promote help-seeking behaviors among men at risk for suicide. Some key initiatives include:

1. **National Suicide Prevention Lifeline:** The National Suicide Prevention Lifeline provides confidential support and crisis

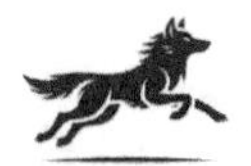

intervention services to individuals in distress. The lifeline is available 24/7 and offers immediate assistance to individuals at risk of suicide.

2. **Community-Based Mental Health Programs:** Community-based mental health programs, such as crisis centers, support groups, and counseling services, provide valuable support and resources to individuals at risk of suicide. These programs offer accessible and localized services to help individuals in need.

3. **Public Awareness Campaigns:** Public awareness campaigns, such as the "It's Okay to Talk" campaign and the "Seize the Awkward" campaign, aim to reduce stigma, promote mental health awareness, and encourage individuals to seek help. These campaigns use various media channels, including social media, television, and print, to reach diverse audiences and promote positive mental health messages.

4. **Policy Initiatives:** Policy initiatives that promote mental health awareness, increase access to mental health services, and support mental health research are essential for addressing the suicide crisis. Advocacy for mental health parity, funding for mental health programs, and the implementation of evidence-based policies are critical components of suicide prevention efforts.

Crisis Intervention and Support Services

Crisis intervention and support services are essential for providing immediate assistance to individuals at risk of suicide. These services include:

1. **Crisis Hotlines:** Crisis hotlines, such as the National Suicide Prevention Lifeline and the Veterans Crisis Line, provide immediate support and intervention for individuals in crisis. These hotlines offer confidential and compassionate assistance, helping individuals navigate their mental health challenges and access appropriate resources.

2. **Mobile Crisis Teams:** Mobile crisis teams, composed of mental health professionals, provide on-site crisis intervention and support to individuals in distress. These teams can respond to crisis situations, conduct assessments, and connect individuals with appropriate mental health services.

3. **Crisis Stabilization Units:** Crisis stabilization units provide short-term, intensive mental health care for individuals experiencing a mental health crisis. These units offer a safe and supportive environment for individuals to stabilize and receive treatment before transitioning to outpatient care.

4. **Peer Support Services:** Peer support services, where individuals with lived experience provide support and guidance to others facing similar challenges, are valuable components of crisis intervention. Peer support can help reduce feelings of isolation, build trust, and promote hope and recovery.

Role of Healthcare Providers and Policymakers

Healthcare providers and policymakers play a crucial role in suicide prevention efforts. Their responsibilities include:

1. **Screening and Assessment:** Healthcare providers should conduct regular screenings and assessments for suicide risk, particularly among high-risk populations such as men with mental health disorders, substance use disorders, and veterans. Early identification of suicide risk allows for timely intervention and support.

2. **Integrated Care:** Integrating mental health care into primary care settings can help improve access to mental health services and reduce stigma. Healthcare providers should work collaboratively to address the mental health needs of their patients and provide comprehensive care.

3. **Training and Education:** Healthcare providers should receive training and education on recognizing and responding to suicide risk. Training programs should emphasize the importance of compassionate and non-judgmental care, as well as the use of evidence-based interventions.

4. **Policy Advocacy:** Policymakers should advocate for policies that promote mental health awareness, increase access to mental health services, and support suicide prevention research. Implementing policies that address economic stress, substance use, and access to lethal means are essential components of suicide prevention efforts.

Public Awareness Campaigns and Education

Public awareness campaigns and education initiatives are essential for reducing stigma, promoting mental health awareness, and encouraging help-seeking behaviors. These efforts include:

1. **Media Campaigns:** Media campaigns that promote positive mental health messages and encourage individuals to seek help can help reduce stigma and increase awareness. These campaigns should use diverse media channels to reach a wide audience and promote mental health literacy.

2. **Educational Programs:** Educational programs in schools, workplaces, and community organizations can help raise awareness about mental health and suicide prevention. These programs should provide information on recognizing the signs of suicide risk, accessing mental health resources, and supporting individuals in distress.

3. **Community Engagement:** Engaging communities in suicide prevention efforts is essential for building a supportive and connected environment. Community events, workshops, and support groups can help promote mental health awareness and provide opportunities for individuals to connect and support one another.

4. **Advocacy and Partnerships:** Advocacy efforts and partnerships with mental health organizations, community leaders, and policymakers are critical for promoting mental health awareness and supporting suicide prevention initiatives. Collaborating with diverse stakeholders can help create a comprehensive and coordinated approach to suicide prevention.

The high suicide rates among men in the United States represent a significant public health crisis that requires urgent attention. Understanding the factors that contribute to this crisis and implementing effective prevention strategies are essential steps toward reducing suicide rates and promoting mental health and well-being.

By addressing the unique challenges faced by men, including mental health disorders, substance abuse, social isolation, economic stress, and access to lethal means, we can develop targeted interventions to support men's mental health and prevent suicide. Collaboration among healthcare providers, policymakers, mental health organizations, and communities is essential for creating a supportive and connected environment that promotes mental health and prevents suicide.

The next chapter will explore the mental health issues specific to military veterans in greater detail, examining the unique challenges they face and the programs and initiatives designed to support their mental health and well-being.

Chapter 7

Mental Health Issues Among Military Veterans

Introduction to Veterans' Mental Health

Military veterans represent a unique population with distinct mental health needs. The experiences and challenges associated with military service, including combat exposure, physical injuries, and the transition to civilian life, can have a profound impact on veterans' mental health. Addressing these mental health issues is essential for supporting the well-being of veterans and honoring their service and sacrifice.

The mental health of veterans is a critical concern that demands focused attention and resources. This chapter explores the prevalence of mental health disorders among veterans, the unique factors contributing to these issues, and the challenges veterans face in accessing care. By understanding these factors and highlighting effective programs and initiatives, we can work towards improving mental health outcomes for veterans.

Prevalence of Mental Health Disorders Among Veterans

Statistics on PTSD, Depression, Anxiety, and Other Disorders

Mental health disorders are prevalent among military veterans, with conditions such as post-traumatic stress disorder (PTSD), depression, and anxiety being particularly common. According to the Department of Veterans Affairs (VA), approximately 11-20% of veterans who served in Operations Iraqi Freedom (OIF) and Enduring Freedom (OEF) have PTSD in a given year. Among Vietnam War veterans, the prevalence of PTSD is estimated to be around 30%.

Depression and anxiety are also significant concerns for veterans. Studies have shown that veterans are at an increased risk for these mental health disorders compared to the general population. The National Center for PTSD reports that about 14% of veterans experience major depressive disorder, and anxiety disorders are prevalent among veterans, with many experiencing generalized anxiety disorder, panic disorder, and social anxiety disorder.

Substance use disorders, including alcohol and drug addiction, are prevalent among veterans. The Substance Abuse and Mental Health Services Administration (SAMHSA) reports that veterans are more likely to misuse alcohol and drugs compared to their civilian counterparts. Substance use disorders often co-occur with other mental health conditions, exacerbating the overall mental health challenges faced by veterans.

The impact of these mental health disorders on veterans' lives can be profound, affecting their relationships, employment, physical health, and overall quality of life. Addressing these mental health issues is essential for supporting veterans' well-being and helping them lead fulfilling lives.

Analysis of the Impact of Combat and Military Service on Mental Health

The experiences associated with combat and military service can have a significant impact on veterans' mental health. Exposure to combat, witnessing traumatic events, and the constant threat of danger can lead to the development of PTSD and other mental health disorders. The psychological toll of combat is often compounded by physical injuries, loss of comrades, and the stress of military operations.

PTSD is one of the most well-documented mental health conditions associated with combat exposure. Symptoms of PTSD can include flashbacks, nightmares, hypervigilance, and emotional numbness. These symptoms can be debilitating and interfere with daily functioning, relationships, and overall well-being.

The transition to civilian life can also be challenging for veterans and can contribute to mental health issues. The loss of military structure, identity, and camaraderie can lead to feelings of isolation, depression, and anxiety. Veterans may also face difficulties in finding employment, securing housing, and accessing healthcare, which can exacerbate mental health challenges.

The impact of combat and military service on mental health extends beyond PTSD and includes a range of conditions such as depression, anxiety, and substance use disorders. Addressing the mental health needs of veterans requires a comprehensive approach that considers the unique experiences and challenges associated with military service.

Unique Factors Contributing to Veterans' Mental Health Issues

Combat-Related Trauma and PTSD

Combat-related trauma is one of the most significant factors contributing to mental health issues among veterans. The experiences of combat, including exposure to violence, injury, and the death of comrades, can lead to the development of PTSD and other trauma-related conditions. The intensity and frequency of combat exposure can exacerbate the severity of these mental health issues.

PTSD is characterized by symptoms such as intrusive memories, flashbacks, nightmares, hypervigilance, and emotional numbness. Veterans with PTSD may experience difficulty in functioning in daily life, maintaining relationships, and engaging in activities they once enjoyed. The chronic nature of PTSD can lead to long-term mental health challenges and significantly impact overall well-being.

The stigma associated with PTSD and other combat-related mental health conditions can prevent veterans from seeking help. Veterans may fear being perceived as weak or unfit for duty, leading to reluctance to disclose their struggles and access mental health services. Addressing this stigma and promoting a culture of acceptance and support within the military and veteran communities is essential for encouraging veterans to seek help.

The impact of PTSD on veterans is not limited to psychological symptoms. It can also lead to physical health problems, such as cardiovascular disease, chronic pain, and immune system dysfunction. The interplay between mental and physical health highlights the importance of a holistic approach to treating PTSD and supporting veterans' overall well-being.

Transition to Civilian Life and Loss of Military Identity

The transition from military to civilian life can be a significant source of stress and mental health challenges for veterans. The loss of military structure, purpose, and identity can lead to feelings of isolation, depression, and anxiety. Veterans may struggle to find a new sense of purpose and belonging in civilian life, which can exacerbate mental health issues.

The challenges of reintegration into civilian life can include difficulties in finding employment, securing housing, and accessing healthcare. Veterans may also face challenges in building and maintaining social connections, leading to feelings of loneliness and isolation. The loss of the camaraderie and support network provided by the military can further contribute to mental health challenges.

Support services and programs that assist veterans in the transition to civilian life are essential for promoting mental health and well-being. These programs can provide resources, counseling, and support to help veterans navigate the challenges of reintegration and find a new sense of purpose and identity.

Programs such as the VA's Transition Assistance Program (TAP) and nonprofit initiatives like "Hire Heroes USA" offer valuable resources and support to veterans as they transition to civilian employment. These programs provide job training, resume building, and networking opportunities to help veterans secure meaningful employment and rebuild their sense of identity and purpose.

Physical Injuries and Chronic Pain

Physical injuries and chronic pain are common among veterans and can have a significant impact on mental health. Many veterans live with physical injuries sustained during military service, including traumatic brain injuries (TBI), amputations, and musculoskeletal injuries. Chronic pain associated with these injuries can lead to mental health issues such as depression and anxiety.

The experience of chronic pain can be debilitating and affect all aspects of a veteran's life, including their ability to work, engage in activities, and maintain relationships. The physical limitations imposed by chronic pain can lead to feelings of frustration, hopelessness, and isolation, further exacerbating mental health challenges.

Comprehensive pain management and rehabilitation services are essential for addressing the physical and mental health needs of veterans with chronic pain. Integrating mental health care with pain management can help address the complex interplay between physical and mental health issues and improve overall well-being.

Programs that provide holistic pain management, including physical therapy, occupational therapy, and cognitive-behavioral therapy (CBT), can be effective in addressing both the physical and psychological aspects of chronic pain. Additionally, support groups for veterans with chronic pain can provide valuable peer support and reduce feelings of isolation.

Substance Abuse and Addiction

Substance abuse and addiction are significant concerns among veterans and are closely linked to mental health issues. Veterans may turn to alcohol and drugs as a way to cope with the stress, trauma, and mental health challenges associated with military service. Substance use can provide temporary relief from emotional pain but can lead to long-term mental health deterioration and increased suicide risk.

The prevalence of substance use disorders among veterans is higher than in the general population. The use of alcohol, prescription medications, and illicit drugs can lead to a cycle of addiction, mental health issues, and social and economic consequences. Veterans with co-occurring substance use and mental health disorders face additional challenges in accessing and receiving effective treatment.

Addressing substance abuse and addiction among veterans requires comprehensive and integrated treatment approaches that address both substance use and mental health issues. Providing access to evidence-based treatment, peer support, and recovery programs is essential for supporting veterans in overcoming addiction and improving mental health.

Veterans Treatment Courts (VTCs) are an innovative approach to addressing substance abuse and mental health issues among veterans involved in the criminal justice system. VTCs provide a specialized court docket that offers treatment and support services as an alternative to incarceration, helping veterans access the care they need and reduce recidivism.

Stigma and Barriers to Seeking Help

Stigma and barriers to seeking help are significant challenges that prevent veterans from accessing mental health care. The stigma associated with mental health issues in the military and veteran communities can lead to reluctance to disclose mental health struggles and seek treatment. Veterans may fear being perceived as weak, unfit for duty, or burdensome to their families and communities.

Barriers to seeking help can include a lack of awareness about available mental health services, concerns about confidentiality, and logistical challenges such as transportation and scheduling. Veterans living in rural or remote areas may face additional barriers to accessing care due to limited availability of mental health providers and services.

Addressing stigma and barriers to seeking help requires a multifaceted approach that includes public awareness campaigns, education, and advocacy. Promoting a culture of acceptance and support within the military and veteran communities, providing information about available services, and reducing logistical barriers are essential steps in encouraging veterans to seek help and access mental health care.

Programs like the VA's "Make the Connection" campaign aim to reduce stigma and promote help-seeking behaviors by sharing personal stories of veterans who have successfully navigated mental health challenges. These stories can help normalize the experience of seeking help and encourage other veterans to access the care they need.

Challenges in Accessing Mental Health Care

Availability and Accessibility of Services

The availability and accessibility of mental health services are significant challenges for many veterans. In some areas, particularly rural and underserved communities, there is a shortage of mental health providers and services. Long wait times for appointments, limited availability of specialized care, and geographic isolation can prevent veterans from receiving timely and appropriate mental health care.

The VA provides a range of mental health services to veterans, but accessing these services can be challenging for some veterans due to logistical barriers such as transportation and scheduling. Veterans may also face challenges in navigating the VA system and understanding their eligibility for services.

Increasing the availability and accessibility of mental health services requires investment in the mental health workforce, expanding telehealth services, and integrating mental health care into primary care settings. Providing transportation assistance and flexible scheduling options can also help reduce barriers to accessing care.

The VA's Office of Rural Health (ORH) works to improve access to care for veterans living in rural areas by expanding telehealth services, providing transportation support, and partnering with community-based providers.

These efforts are essential for ensuring that rural veterans receive the mental health care they need.

Cultural Competence and Veteran-Specific Care

Cultural competence and veteran-specific care are essential for providing effective mental health services to veterans. Mental health providers who understand the unique experiences and challenges of military service can provide more effective and compassionate care. Culturally competent care includes understanding the military culture, recognizing the impact of combat and trauma, and addressing the specific needs of veterans.

Veterans may feel more comfortable seeking help from providers who have experience working with military and veteran populations. Providing training and education for mental health providers on the unique needs of veterans can help improve the quality of care and increase veterans' willingness to seek help.

Integrating veteran-specific care into mental health services can include providing specialized programs for PTSD, substance use disorders, and other conditions prevalent among veterans. Peer support programs that connect veterans with others who have shared experiences can also provide valuable support and reduce feelings of isolation.

The VA's National Center for PTSD offers resources and training for mental health providers to improve their understanding of PTSD and enhance their ability to provide effective care to veterans. This training includes evidence-based treatments such as Prolonged Exposure (PE) therapy and Cognitive Processing Therapy (CPT), which have been shown to be effective in treating PTSD.

Financial and Logistical Barriers

Financial and logistical barriers can prevent veterans from accessing mental health care. The cost of mental health services, including therapy and medication, can be prohibitive for some veterans, particularly those without adequate insurance coverage. High out-of-pocket costs and limited coverage for mental health services can prevent veterans from seeking the care they need.

Logistical barriers, such as transportation, scheduling, and childcare, can also hinder access to mental health services. Veterans living in rural or remote areas may face additional challenges due to limited availability of providers and services. Addressing these barriers requires comprehensive strategies that include financial assistance, transportation support, and flexible scheduling options.

The VA provides mental health services at no cost to eligible veterans, but navigating the VA system and understanding eligibility can be challenging. Providing clear information and assistance with navigating the VA system can help veterans access the services they need.

Programs like the VA's Veterans Transportation Service (VTS) offer free transportation to and from VA medical appointments for veterans who face transportation challenges. This service is essential for ensuring that veterans can access the care they need, particularly those living in rural or underserved areas.

Impact of Rural Living and Geographic Isolation

Veterans living in rural areas face unique challenges in accessing mental health care. Geographic isolation, limited availability of mental health providers, and transportation challenges can prevent rural veterans from receiving timely and appropriate care. Rural veterans may also experience increased social isolation and limited access to support networks, further exacerbating mental health challenges.

Expanding telehealth services is a critical strategy for addressing the mental health needs of rural veterans. Telehealth can provide convenient and accessible mental health care, reducing barriers related to transportation and geographic location. Integrating telehealth services into VA and community-based programs can help ensure that rural veterans receive the care they need.

Community-based initiatives that engage local organizations, faith-based groups, and community leaders can also help support the mental health needs of rural veterans. These initiatives can provide resources, support, and opportunities for social connection, helping to reduce feelings of isolation and promote mental well-being.

The VA's Rural Health Resource Centers (RHRCs) work to improve access to care for rural veterans by conducting research, developing innovative care models, and providing training and resources to rural healthcare providers. These efforts are essential for ensuring that rural veterans receive high-quality mental health care.

Programs and Initiatives Supporting Veterans' Mental Health

Overview of VA Mental Health Services

The Department of Veterans Affairs (VA) provides a comprehensive range of mental health services to veterans. These services include counseling, therapy, medication management, and specialized programs for conditions such as PTSD, depression, anxiety, and substance use disorders. The VA also offers inpatient and outpatient care, crisis intervention services, and support for the transition to civilian life.

The VA's mental health services are designed to be veteran-centered and culturally competent, addressing the unique needs and experiences of veterans. The VA provides care through its network of medical centers, outpatient clinics, Vet Centers, and community-based programs. Telehealth services have also been expanded to increase access to care, particularly for veterans in rural and underserved areas.

The VA's commitment to continuous improvement and innovation in mental health care is reflected in its research initiatives and partnerships with academic institutions and community organizations. The VA conducts research on the effectiveness of mental health treatments and develops evidence-based practices to improve care and outcomes for veterans.

The VA's Whole Health approach to care emphasizes the importance of holistic well-being, incorporating physical, mental, and spiritual health into treatment plans. This approach empowers veterans to take an active role in their health and well-being, promoting resilience and improving overall quality of life.

Community-Based Programs and Nonprofit Organizations

In addition to the VA, community-based programs and nonprofit organizations play a vital role in supporting veterans' mental health. These programs provide a range of services, including counseling, peer support, crisis intervention, and assistance with the transition to civilian life. Community-based programs often offer more flexible and accessible services, particularly for veterans who may face barriers to accessing VA care.

Non-profit organizations such as Wounded Warrior Project, Team Red, White & Blue, Veterans of Foreign Wars (VFW), and MENtality Matters provide valuable support and resources to veterans. These organizations offer programs that promote mental health, physical wellness, and social connection, helping veterans build resilience and improve overall well-being.

Collaboration between the VA, community-based programs, and non-profit organizations is essential for providing comprehensive and coordinated care to veterans. These partnerships can help address gaps in services, increase access to care, and provide a more holistic approach to supporting veterans' mental health.

Programs like Wounded Warrior Project's "Warrior Care Network" provide intensive outpatient mental health care for veterans with PTSD, TBI, and other conditions. This program partners with academic medical centers to offer evidence-based treatment and support, helping veterans achieve lasting recovery.

Innovative Approaches and Telehealth

Innovative approaches to mental health care are essential for addressing the unique needs of veterans and improving access to services. Telehealth has become an increasingly important tool for providing mental health care, particularly during the COVID-19 pandemic. Telehealth services can offer convenient and accessible care, reducing barriers related to transportation, scheduling, and geographic location.

The VA has expanded its telehealth services to provide virtual counseling, therapy, and medication management to veterans. Telehealth platforms allow veterans to connect with mental health providers from the comfort of their homes, increasing access to care and reducing the stigma associated with seeking help.

Other innovative approaches to mental health care for veterans include the use of technology-based interventions, such as mobile apps and online support groups. These tools can provide additional support and resources to veterans, helping them manage their mental health and connect with others who share similar experiences.

The VA's "Mobile Vet Centers" provide outreach and counseling services to veterans in rural and underserved areas. These mobile units are equipped with private counseling spaces and technology for telehealth services, bringing mental health care directly to veterans who may face barriers to accessing traditional care.

Role of Peer Support and Veteran Advocacy Groups

Peer support and veteran advocacy groups play a critical role in supporting veterans' mental health. Peer support programs connect veterans with others who have shared experiences, providing valuable social connection, emotional support, and practical guidance. Veterans who have successfully navigated mental health challenges and are willing to share their experiences can serve as role models and mentors for others.

Veteran advocacy groups, such as the American Legion and Iraq and Afghanistan Veterans of America (IAVA), advocate for policies and programs that support veterans' mental health and well-being. These organizations work to raise awareness about veterans' mental health issues, promote access to care, and advocate for policy changes to improve services and support for veterans.

By providing peer support, advocacy, and resources, these groups help build a supportive and connected veteran community. Their efforts contribute to reducing stigma, increasing access to care, and promoting mental health and well-being among veterans.

Programs like the VA's "Peer Support Specialist" initiative train veterans with lived experience in mental health recovery to provide peer support services to other veterans. These specialists offer valuable insights and support, helping veterans navigate the challenges of mental health recovery and connect with resources and services.

The mental health challenges faced by military veterans are complex and multifaceted, requiring targeted and comprehensive interventions. By understanding the unique factors contributing to veterans' mental health issues and addressing the barriers to accessing care, we can work towards improving mental health outcomes for veterans.

Programs and initiatives that provide comprehensive and accessible mental health care, promote social connections, and support the transition to civilian life are essential for supporting veterans' well-being. Collaboration between the VA, community-based programs, nonprofit organizations, and veteran advocacy groups is critical for providing coordinated and effective care.

The next chapter will explore the current policies related to mental health care for men and veterans, analyzing their effectiveness and proposing changes to improve access and outcomes.

Chapter 8

Analysis of Current Mental Health Policies for Men and Veterans

Introduction to Mental Health Policies

Mental health policies play a crucial role in shaping the availability, accessibility, and quality of mental health care for individuals. For men and veterans, effective mental health policies are essential for addressing unique challenges and ensuring that they receive the support and care they need. This chapter explores current mental health policies in the United States, evaluates their effectiveness, identifies gaps and challenges, and proposes changes to improve access and outcomes.

Policymakers, mental health professionals, and advocacy groups all have a critical role in shaping mental health policies. By understanding the strengths and weaknesses of existing policies and advocating for necessary reforms, we can work towards a more inclusive and effective mental health care system for men and veterans.

Current Mental Health Policies for Men

Analysis of Policies at the Federal, State, and Local Levels

Mental health policies for men in the United States are shaped by a combination of federal, state, and local initiatives. At the federal level, key policies include the Mental Health Parity and Addiction Equity Act (MHPAEA), the Affordable Care Act (ACA), and the Substance Abuse and Mental Health Services Administration (SAMHSA) programs. These policies aim to increase access to mental health services, promote parity between mental and physical health care, and provide funding for mental health initiatives.

The MHPAEA, enacted in 2008, requires that health insurance plans offer mental health and substance use disorder benefits that are no more restrictive than medical and surgical benefits. This legislation has been instrumental in improving access to mental health care for men by reducing financial barriers and promoting equitable coverage. The ACA further expanded access to mental health care by requiring most insurance plans to cover mental health services as essential health benefits.

At the state level, policies vary widely, with some states implementing comprehensive mental health initiatives and others lacking adequate resources and support. State mental health policies can include funding for community mental health services, crisis intervention programs, and initiatives to reduce stigma and promote mental health awareness. Local governments also play a role in mental health policy by implementing community-based programs and services that address the specific needs of their populations.

For example, California's Mental Health Services Act (MHSA), funded by a 1% tax on incomes over $1 million, provides substantial resources for mental health programs across the state. This act has enabled the development of innovative programs and services, including crisis intervention, early psychosis treatment, and community-based support.

Workplace mental health policies are another important aspect of mental health care for men. Employers can implement policies that promote mental health awareness, provide access to employee assistance programs (EAPs), and support work-life balance. Workplace policies that prioritize mental health can help reduce stigma, encourage help-seeking behaviors, and improve overall well-being for employees.

Impact of the Mental Health Parity and Addiction Equity Act (MHPAEA)

The Mental Health Parity and Addiction Equity Act (MHPAEA) has had a significant impact on mental health care in the United States. By requiring parity between mental health and physical health benefits, the MHPAEA has reduced financial barriers to mental health care and increased access to necessary services. The act applies to employer-sponsored health plans, individual and small group plans, and Medicaid managed care plans.

The MHPAEA has helped to reduce disparities in mental health care access and ensure that individuals, including men, receive comprehensive coverage for mental health services. However, challenges remain in fully implementing and enforcing parity requirements. Some insurance plans continue to impose restrictions on mental health benefits, such as limited provider networks and prior authorization requirements, which can hinder access to care.

Ongoing efforts to strengthen and enforce parity laws are essential for ensuring that all individuals have access to equitable mental health care. Policymakers, mental health professionals, and advocacy groups must work together to address gaps in implementation and advocate for policies that promote true parity between mental and physical health care.

One significant challenge is the variability in enforcement across states. Some states have implemented robust parity enforcement mechanisms, while others lack the resources or political will to fully enforce the law. The federal government can play a critical role in supporting state efforts through funding, technical assistance, and oversight.

Evaluation of Workplace Mental Health Policies

Workplace mental health policies play a crucial role in supporting the mental health and well-being of employees. Effective workplace policies can help reduce stigma, encourage help-seeking behaviors, and provide access to mental health resources and support. Key components of workplace mental health policies include:

1. **Employee Assistance Programs (EAPs):** EAPs provide confidential counseling and support services to employees experiencing mental health issues, stress, or other personal challenges. EAPs can offer short-term counseling, referrals to mental health providers, and resources for managing work-life balance.

2. **Mental Health Awareness and Education:** Workplace policies that promote mental health awareness and education can help reduce stigma and encourage employees to seek help. Training programs for managers and employees can provide information on recognizing signs of mental health issues, accessing resources, and supporting colleagues.

3. **Flexible Work Arrangements:** Flexible work arrangements, such as remote work, flexible hours, and job-sharing, can help employees manage stress and maintain a healthy work-life balance. Policies that support flexible work arrangements can improve overall well-being and reduce the risk of burnout.

4. **Supportive Work Environment:** Creating a supportive work environment involves fostering a culture of openness and acceptance, where employees feel comfortable discussing mental health issues and seeking help. Employers can promote a supportive environment by providing mental health resources, offering regular check-ins, and encouraging open communication.

While many employers have implemented workplace mental health policies, challenges remain in ensuring that these policies are effective and accessible to all employees. Employers must continually assess and improve their mental health policies, provide ongoing training and support, and create a culture that prioritizes mental health and well-being.

Examples of successful workplace mental health initiatives include the "Mind Matters" program at Johnson & Johnson, which provides mental health resources, training, and support to employees. Another example is the "Employee Well-being Initiative" at Google, which offers a range of mental health services, including on-site counseling, mindfulness programs, and resilience training.

Current Mental Health Policies for Veterans

Overview of VA Mental Health Policies and Programs

The Department of Veterans Affairs (VA) is responsible for providing comprehensive mental health services to veterans. VA mental health policies and programs are designed to address the unique needs of veterans, including those related to combat exposure, trauma, and the transition to civilian life. Key components of VA mental health policies and programs include:

1. **VA Medical Centers and Clinics:** The VA operates a network of medical centers and outpatient clinics that provide a wide range of mental health services, including counseling, therapy, medication management, and specialized programs for PTSD, depression, and substance use disorders.

2. **Vet Centers:** Vet Centers provide readjustment counseling and support to veterans and their families. These centers offer individual and group counseling, crisis intervention, and assistance with navigating VA services.

3. **Telehealth Services:** The VA has expanded its telehealth services to provide virtual mental health care to veterans, particularly those in rural and underserved areas. Telehealth platforms allow veterans to connect with mental health providers from the comfort of their homes, increasing access to care and reducing barriers.

4. **Crisis Intervention and Support:** The Veterans Crisis Line provides confidential support and crisis intervention services to veterans and their families. The hotline is available 24/7 and offers immediate assistance to veterans in crisis.

5. **Specialized Programs:** The VA offers specialized programs for veterans with PTSD, substance use disorders, traumatic brain injuries (TBI), and other conditions. These programs provide evidence-based treatments and support to help veterans manage their mental health and achieve recovery.

The VA's commitment to providing veteran-centered and culturally competent care is reflected in its policies and programs. The VA continuously evaluates and improves its mental health services to ensure that they meet the needs of veterans and support their overall well-being.

The VA's "Whole Health" approach emphasizes the importance of addressing physical, mental, and social factors that impact health. This holistic approach empowers veterans to take an active role in their health and well-being, promoting resilience and improving overall quality of life.

Analysis of the Veterans Health Administration (VHA) Policies

The Veterans Health Administration (VHA) is the largest integrated healthcare system in the United States and plays a critical role in providing mental health care to veterans. VHA policies are designed to ensure that veterans receive high-quality, accessible, and comprehensive mental health services. Key aspects of VHA policies include:

1. **Integrated Mental Health Care:** VHA policies emphasize the integration of mental health care into primary care settings. This approach ensures that veterans receive holistic care that addresses both their physical and mental health needs. Integrated care models promote early identification and intervention for mental health issues and improve overall health outcomes.

2. **Evidence-Based Practices:** The VHA is committed to using evidence-based practices in its mental health services. This commitment includes implementing treatments that have been proven effective through research, such as Cognitive Behavioral Therapy (CBT), Prolonged Exposure (PE) therapy, and Cognitive Processing Therapy (CPT) for PTSD.

3. **Veteran-Centered Care:** VHA policies prioritize veteran-centered care, which involves tailoring services to meet the unique needs and preferences of veterans. This approach includes involving veterans in their treatment plans, providing culturally competent care, and addressing the social determinants of health that impact mental well-being.

4. **Access to Care:** The VHA is dedicated to improving access to mental health care for all veterans. This commitment includes expanding telehealth services, increasing the availability of mental health providers, and reducing wait times for appointments. The VHA also provides transportation assistance and support to help veterans access care.

5. **Research and Innovation:** The VHA conducts research on mental health issues affecting veterans and develops innovative care models to improve outcomes. This research includes studying the effectiveness of treatments, identifying risk factors for mental health issues, and developing new interventions.

The VHA's policies and programs reflect a commitment to providing comprehensive and high-quality mental health care to veterans. Ongoing evaluation and improvement of these policies are essential for addressing the evolving needs of veterans and ensuring that they receive the support and care they deserve.

The VHA's "Primary Care-Mental Health Integration" (PC-MHI) program exemplifies its commitment to integrated care. This program embeds mental health professionals within primary care teams, allowing for immediate consultation and coordinated care for veterans with mental health concerns.

Evaluation of Recent Legislative Initiatives

Recent legislative initiatives have aimed to improve mental health care for veterans and address the unique challenges they face. Key legislative initiatives include:

1. **Commander John Scott Hannon Veterans Mental Health Care Improvement Act:** Enacted in 2020, this legislation aims to improve mental health care for veterans by expanding access to services, increasing funding for mental health programs, and promoting innovative care models. Key provisions of the act include expanding telehealth services, increasing mental health provider training, and supporting community-based programs.

2. **VA MISSION Act:** The VA MISSION Act, enacted in 2018, aims to improve access to care for veterans by expanding eligibility for community care, increasing funding for the VA, and improving the VA's ability to recruit and retain healthcare providers. The act includes provisions to enhance mental health care for veterans, such as increasing access to telehealth services and improving care coordination.

3. **Clay Hunt SAV Act:** The Clay Hunt Suicide Prevention for American Veterans (SAV) Act, enacted in 2015, aims to reduce veteran suicide by improving access to mental health care and promoting community-based support. Key provisions of the act include increasing funding for mental health programs, expanding peer support services, and improving the VA's ability to track and monitor suicide prevention efforts.

4. **Veterans' ACCESS Act:** This act focuses on increasing access to mental health care for veterans by expanding telehealth services, improving care coordination, and providing additional funding for mental health programs. The act also includes provisions to support community-based mental health initiatives and promote collaboration between the VA and local organizations.

These legislative initiatives reflect a commitment to improving mental health care for veterans and addressing the unique challenges they face. Ongoing advocacy and support for these initiatives are essential for ensuring that veterans receive the comprehensive and high-quality care they need.

The Commander John Scott Hannon Veterans Mental Health Care Improvement Act, for example, includes provisions for the development of a "Precision Medicine Initiative" for veterans with PTSD. This initiative aims to tailor treatments to the individual needs of veterans, improving outcomes and reducing the burden of PTSD.

Gaps and Challenges in Existing Policies

Identification of Gaps in Coverage and Accessibility

Despite significant progress in mental health policy, gaps in coverage and accessibility remain. Key gaps include:

1. **Insurance Coverage:** While the MHPAEA has improved access to mental health care, some insurance plans continue to impose restrictions on mental health benefits, such as limited provider networks and prior authorization requirements. These restrictions can hinder access to care and create financial barriers for individuals seeking mental health services.

2. **Access to Care:** Geographic disparities in access to mental health care persist, particularly in rural and underserved areas. The shortage of mental health providers in these areas can result in long wait times for appointments and limited availability of specialized care.

3. **Cultural Competence:** There is a need for increased cultural competence among mental health providers to address the unique needs of diverse populations, including men and veterans. Culturally competent care involves understanding and addressing the cultural, social, and linguistic factors that impact mental health.

4. **Coordination of Care:** Gaps in care coordination can result in fragmented and inconsistent mental health services. Improved care coordination is essential for ensuring that individuals receive comprehensive and continuous care, particularly for those with complex mental health needs.

5. **Stigma and Barriers to Seeking Help:** Stigma remains a significant barrier to accessing mental health care for many individuals. Efforts to reduce stigma and promote help-seeking behaviors are essential

for improving access to care and supporting mental health and well-being.

6. **Barriers for Veterans Transitioning to Civilian Life:** Veterans often face unique challenges during their transition to civilian life, including difficulties in finding employment, securing housing, and accessing healthcare. These challenges can exacerbate mental health issues and create additional barriers to accessing care.

Addressing these gaps requires targeted policy reforms, increased funding for mental health services, and ongoing advocacy and support from policy-makers, mental health professionals, and advocacy groups.

Challenges in Policy Implementation and Enforcement

Challenges in policy implementation and enforcement can hinder the effectiveness of mental health policies. Key challenges include:

1. **Variability in State Policies:** The variability in mental health policies across states can result in disparities in access to care and quality of services. Some states have implemented comprehensive mental health initiatives, while others lack adequate resources and support.

2. **Resource Limitations:** Limited funding and resources for mental health services can impact the ability to implement and enforce policies effectively. Resource limitations can result in long wait times, limited availability of services, and reduced access to care.

3. **Provider Shortages:** The shortage of mental health providers, particularly in rural and underserved areas, can hinder access to care and impact the quality of services. Efforts to recruit and retain mental health providers are essential for addressing provider shortages and improving access to care.

4. **Complexity of the Mental Health System:** The complexity of the mental health system can create barriers to accessing care and navigating services. Simplifying the system and improving care coordination are essential for ensuring that individuals receive timely and appropriate care.

5. **Monitoring and Evaluation:** Effective policy implementation requires ongoing monitoring and evaluation to assess the impact of policies and identify areas for improvement. Developing robust

monitoring and evaluation systems is essential for ensuring that policies achieve their intended outcomes.

Addressing these challenges requires a coordinated effort from policy-makers, mental health professionals, and advocacy groups to ensure that policies are effectively implemented and enforced.

Impact of Social Determinants of Health on Policy Effectiveness

Social determinants of health, such as socioeconomic status, education, housing, and access to healthcare, play a significant role in shaping mental health outcomes. Addressing these social determinants is essential for improving the effectiveness of mental health policies and ensuring that all individuals have access to the care and support they need.

Key social determinants of health that impact mental health policy effectiveness include:

1. **Economic Stability:** Financial stress and economic instability can exacerbate mental health issues and create barriers to accessing care. Policies that promote economic stability, such as job training programs, financial assistance, and affordable housing, can improve mental health outcomes and support overall well-being.

2. **Education:** Education plays a critical role in shaping mental health outcomes. Policies that promote mental health education and awareness in schools can help reduce stigma, encourage help-seeking behaviors, and provide students with the tools to manage their mental health.

3. **Healthcare Access:** Access to affordable and high-quality healthcare is essential for supporting mental health. Policies that expand healthcare access, such as Medicaid expansion and community health centers, can improve mental health outcomes and reduce disparities in care.

4. **Social and Community Support:** Social connections and community support are important for mental health and well-being. Policies that promote social and community engagement, such as community centers, support groups, and peer support programs, can reduce isolation and provide valuable resources and support.

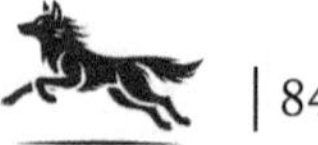

5. **Environmental Factors:** Environmental factors, such as housing quality and neighborhood safety, can impact mental health outcomes. Policies that address environmental determinants, such as affordable housing initiatives and community development programs, can improve mental health and overall quality of life.

Addressing the social determinants of health requires a comprehensive approach that includes policy reforms, community-based initiatives, and collaboration between multiple sectors. By addressing these determinants, we can improve the effectiveness of mental health policies and promote mental health and well-being for all individuals.

Proposed Changes to Improve Mental Health Policies

Recommendations for Policy Reforms

To improve mental health policies for men and veterans, the following recommendations are proposed:

1. **Strengthen Parity Laws:** Strengthen and enforce parity laws to ensure that mental health benefits are equivalent to physical health benefits. This includes addressing gaps in coverage, reducing restrictions on mental health services, and increasing transparency and accountability.
2. **Expand Access to Care:** Expand access to mental health care by increasing funding for mental health services, expanding telehealth services, and addressing provider shortages. This includes investing in the mental health workforce, providing incentives for mental health providers to work in underserved areas, and increasing support for community-based programs.
3. **Promote Cultural Competence:** Promote cultural competence among mental health providers to address the unique needs of diverse populations. This includes providing training and education on cultural competence, developing culturally tailored interventions, and increasing the availability of culturally competent providers.
4. **Improve Care Coordination:** Improve care coordination to ensure that individuals receive comprehensive and continuous

care. This includes developing integrated care models, enhancing communication between providers, and providing support for care coordination.

5. **Address Social Determinants of Health:** Address the social determinants of health that impact mental health outcomes. This includes promoting economic stability, expanding access to education, improving healthcare access, enhancing social and community support, and addressing environmental factors.

6. **Reduce Stigma:** Implement public awareness campaigns and education initiatives to reduce stigma and promote help-seeking behaviors. This includes sharing personal stories, providing information on mental health resources, and encouraging open conversations about mental health.

7. **Enhance Policy Implementation and Enforcement:** Enhance the implementation and enforcement of mental health policies by providing adequate resources, developing robust monitoring and evaluation systems, and ensuring consistency in policies across states.

8. **Support Veterans Transitioning to Civilian Life:** Provide targeted support for veterans transitioning to civilian life. This includes job training programs, housing assistance, and mental health services to address the unique challenges faced by veterans during this transition.

By implementing these recommendations, we can improve mental health policies for men and veterans and ensure that they receive the support and care they need.

Strategies for Improving Access and Reducing Barriers

To improve access to mental health care and reduce barriers, the following strategies are proposed:

1. **Increase Funding for Mental Health Services:** Increase funding for mental health services to ensure that individuals have access to high-quality and affordable care. This includes funding for community-based programs, telehealth services, and initiatives to address provider shortages.

2. **Expand Telehealth Services:** Expand telehealth services to provide convenient and accessible mental health care. This includes investing in telehealth infrastructure, providing training for providers, and promoting the use of telehealth services among individuals.

3. **Provide Financial Assistance:** Provide financial assistance to individuals to reduce the cost of mental health services. This includes expanding insurance coverage for mental health services, providing subsidies for low-income individuals, and offering financial assistance for out-of-pocket costs.

4. **Enhance Transportation Support:** Enhance transportation support to help individuals access mental health care. This includes providing transportation services, offering transportation vouchers, and partnering with community organizations to provide transportation assistance.

5. **Promote Flexible Scheduling:** Promote flexible scheduling options to accommodate individuals' needs and preferences. This includes offering evening and weekend appointments, providing walk-in services, and allowing for flexible appointment scheduling.

6. **Increase Awareness of Available Services:** Increase awareness of available mental health services and resources. This includes providing information on mental health services through public awareness campaigns, community outreach, and partnerships with local organizations.

7. **Improve Provider Training and Retention:** Implement initiatives to improve training and retention of mental health providers. This includes providing incentives for providers to work in underserved areas, offering loan repayment programs, and providing opportunities for professional development and continuing education.

8. **Enhance Community-Based Support:** Strengthen community-based support systems by investing in local mental health programs, peer support groups, and community centers. These resources can provide valuable support and reduce feelings of isolation.

By implementing these strategies, we can improve access to mental health care and reduce barriers for men and veterans, ensuring that they receive the support and care they need.

The role of Mental Health Professionals and Advocacy Groups in Policy Development Mental health professionals and advocacy groups play a critical role in shaping mental health policy and advocating for necessary reforms. Their involvement is essential for ensuring that policies are evidence-based, effective, and responsive to the needs of individuals. Key roles of mental health professionals and advocacy groups include:

1. **Advocacy and Policy Development:** Mental health professionals and advocacy groups can advocate for policy reforms and contribute to the development of mental health policies. This includes providing expert testimony, participating in policy discussions, and collaborating with policymakers.

2. **Education and Training:** Mental health professionals and advocacy groups can provide education and training to policymakers, healthcare providers, and the public. This includes offering training on best practices, cultural competence, and the social determinants of health that impact mental health outcomes.

3. **Research and Evaluation:** Mental health professionals and advocacy groups can conduct research and evaluation to assess the impact of mental health policies and identify areas for improvement. This includes studying the effectiveness of treatments, identifying risk factors for mental health issues, and developing new interventions.

4. **Community Engagement:** Mental health professionals and advocacy groups can engage with communities to promote mental health awareness, reduce stigma, and provide support and resources. This includes partnering with local organizations, offering community-based programs, and providing peer support.

5. **Collaboration and Partnerships:** Mental health professionals and advocacy groups can collaborate with other stakeholders to develop and implement mental health policies. This includes partnering with healthcare providers, community organizations, and policymakers to ensure a coordinated and comprehensive approach to mental health care.

By actively participating in policy development, education, research, community engagement, and collaboration, mental health professionals and advocacy groups can help shape mental health policies that support the well-being of men and veterans.

Mental health policies play a critical role in shaping the availability, accessibility, and quality of mental health care for men and veterans. While significant progress has been made, gaps and challenges remain. By addressing these gaps, implementing targeted policy reforms, and promoting collaboration and advocacy, we can improve mental health policies and ensure that men and veterans receive the support and care they need.

The next chapter will explore the different types of therapies and treatments available for mental health issues, highlighting their effectiveness and providing recommendations for best practices.

Chapter 9

Types of Therapies and Treatments for Mental Health Issues

Introduction to Therapies and Treatments

Effective mental health treatments are essential for improving the quality of life for individuals experiencing mental health issues. These treatments can help individuals manage symptoms, develop coping strategies, and achieve overall well-being. This chapter explores various types of therapies and treatments available for mental health issues, emphasizing their effectiveness and best practices. It includes an overview of traditional therapies, innovative treatments, pharmacological interventions, and integrative approaches. The chapter provides insights into how these therapies can be tailored to meet the specific needs of men and veterans.

Traditional Therapies

Cognitive Behavioral Therapy (CBT)

Cognitive Behavioral Therapy (CBT) is one of the most widely used and evidence-based treatments for mental health issues. CBT focuses on identifying and changing negative thought patterns and behaviors that contribute to mental health problems. It is effective in treating a range of conditions, including depression, anxiety, PTSD, and substance use disorders.

CBT involves several key components:

1. **Cognitive Restructuring:** Identifying and challenging distorted or irrational thoughts and replacing them with more realistic and positive ones.

2. **Behavioral Activation:** Encouraging engagement in activities that promote pleasure and achievement to combat depression and increase positive experiences.

91

3. **Exposure Therapy:** Gradually confronting feared situations or memories in a controlled and safe environment to reduce anxiety and PTSD symptoms.
4. **Skill Building:** Teaching coping skills, problem-solving techniques, and relaxation strategies to manage stress and improve overall functioning.

CBT is highly structured and typically involves a set number of sessions, making it a practical and time-limited approach. Its emphasis on skill-building and self-help strategies empowers individuals to take an active role in their treatment and maintain improvements over the long term.

CBT can be particularly beneficial for men who may be more comfortable with a structured and goal-oriented approach. The practical and solution-focused nature of CBT aligns with many men's preferences for actionable steps and tangible outcomes.

Psychodynamic Therapy

Psychodynamic Therapy is based on the theories of Freud and other psychoanalysts. It focuses on exploring unconscious processes and unresolved conflicts from the past that influence current behavior and emotions. The goal of psychodynamic therapy is to increase self-awareness and understanding of how past experiences shape present behavior.

Key components of psychodynamic therapy include:
1. **Free Association:** Encouraging patients to speak freely about their thoughts and feelings, allowing unconscious material to emerge.
2. **Transference and Countertransference:** Exploring the patient's relationship patterns with the therapist to gain insights into past relationships and unresolved conflicts.
3. **Interpretation:** Analyzing dreams, fantasies, and behaviors to uncover hidden meanings and unconscious motivations.

Psychodynamic therapy can be particularly effective for individuals with complex and deep-seated emotional issues. It is a longer-term therapy compared to CBT, often requiring months or years of treatment to achieve significant change.

For men who may be less comfortable discussing their emotions, psychodynamic therapy can provide a safe and supportive environment to explore underlying issues at a deeper level. It can help men understand and process emotions that may be influencing their behavior and relationships.

Interpersonal Therapy (IPT)

Interpersonal Therapy (IPT) is a short-term, evidence-based treatment that focuses on improving interpersonal relationships and communication skills. IPT is based on the idea that mental health symptoms are often related to difficulties in relationships and social interactions. It is effective in treating depression, anxiety, and other mood disorders.

Key components of IPT include:

1. **Identifying Interpersonal Issues:** Focusing on specific problem areas, such as role transitions, interpersonal disputes, grief, and social isolation.
2. **Improving Communication Skills:** Teaching effective communication strategies to resolve conflicts and improve relationships.
3. **Building Social Support:** Encouraging the development of a strong social support network to enhance emotional well-being.

IPT typically involves 12-16 weekly sessions and is highly structured. It is particularly effective for individuals experiencing depression related to interpersonal issues or significant life changes.

For men who may struggle with expressing emotions or navigating social interactions, IPT provides practical tools and strategies to improve communication and relationships. It can help men build stronger support networks and improve their ability to cope with stress and emotional challenges.

Family and Couples Therapy

Family and Couples Therapy focuses on improving the functioning and dynamics of relationships within a family or between partners. It is based on the idea that individual mental health issues are often influenced by and impact family and relationship dynamics. Family and couples therapy can be effective in addressing a wide range of mental health issues, including depression, anxiety, substance use disorders, and PTSD.

Key components of family and couples therapy include:

1. **Communication Skills:** Teaching effective communication strategies to enhance understanding and reduce conflict.
2. **Problem-Solving Skills:** Developing collaborative problem-solving approaches to address family or relationship issues.
3. **Family Dynamics:** Exploring and addressing dysfunctional patterns and dynamics within the family or relationship.

Family and couples therapy can be particularly beneficial for individuals experiencing mental health issues that are closely linked to relationship stressors. It provides a supportive environment for all family members or partners to work together towards improved mental health and relationship functioning.

Men may find family and couples therapy helpful in addressing issues related to their roles and responsibilities within the family. It can provide a space to discuss and resolve conflicts, improve communication, and strengthen family bonds.

Innovative Treatments

Eye Movement Desensitization and Reprocessing (EMDR)

Eye Movement Desensitization and Reprocessing (EMDR) is an evidence-based treatment specifically designed to help individuals process and resolve traumatic memories. EMDR is particularly effective in treating PTSD but has also been used to address other mental health conditions, such as anxiety, depression, and phobias.

Key components of EMDR include:

1. **Bilateral Stimulation:** Using eye movements, taps, or auditory tones to facilitate the processing of traumatic memories.
2. **Desensitization:** Gradually reducing the emotional distress associated with traumatic memories through repeated exposure and processing.
3. **Reprocessing:** Helping individuals reframe and integrate traumatic memories into a more adaptive and positive perspective.

EMDR typically involves eight phases of treatment, including history-taking, preparation, assessment, desensitization, installation, body scan, closure, and reevaluation. It is a structured and time-limited therapy that can produce rapid and significant improvements in trauma-related symptoms.

EMDR can be particularly beneficial for veterans and men who have experienced trauma. The structured approach and use of bilateral stimulation can make it easier for individuals to process traumatic memories without becoming overwhelmed by emotion.

Acceptance and Commitment Therapy (ACT)

Acceptance and Commitment Therapy (ACT) is an innovative treatment that combines elements of mindfulness and cognitive-behavioral therapy. ACT focuses on helping individuals accept their thoughts and feelings, commit to values-based actions, and develop psychological flexibility. It is effective in treating a wide range of mental health conditions, including depression, anxiety, PTSD, and chronic pain.

Key components of ACT include:

1. **Acceptance:** Encouraging individuals to accept their thoughts and feelings without judgment or avoidance.
2. **Mindfulness:** Promoting present-moment awareness and mindfulness practices to reduce reactivity and increase psychological flexibility.
3. **Values Clarification:** Helping individuals identify their core values and commit to actions that align with those values.
4. **Cognitive Defusion:** Teaching techniques to reduce the impact of negative thoughts and increase cognitive flexibility.

ACT is a highly flexible and individualized therapy that can be adapted to meet the unique needs of each individual. It emphasizes experiential learning and practical strategies for enhancing well-being and resilience.

For men who may struggle with acceptance and avoidance, ACT provides a framework for understanding and addressing these challenges. The focus on values and committed action can help men align their behaviors with their personal goals and values.

Dialectical Behavior Therapy (DBT)

Dialectical Behavior Therapy (DBT) is an evidence-based treatment originally developed for individuals with borderline personality disorder (BPD). DBT has since been adapted to treat a range of mental health conditions, including depression, anxiety, substance use disorders, and PTSD. DBT combines elements of cognitive-behavioral therapy with mindfulness and acceptance strategies.

Key components of DBT include:

1. **Individual Therapy:** Providing one-on-one sessions to address specific mental health issues and develop coping strategies.
2. **Skills Training Groups:** Teaching skills in mindfulness, emotional regulation, distress tolerance, and interpersonal effectiveness.
3. **Phone Coaching:** Offering real-time support and coaching to help individuals apply DBT skills in everyday situations.
4. **Consultation Teams:** Providing support and supervision for DBT therapists to ensure adherence to the treatment model and address challenges.

DBT is a comprehensive and structured therapy that emphasizes the development of practical skills for managing emotions, improving relationships, and reducing harmful behaviors. It is particularly effective for individuals with severe and complex mental health issues.

Men who may have difficulty with emotional regulation and interpersonal relationships can benefit from DBT's structured approach. The skills training and phone coaching components provide ongoing support and reinforcement of therapeutic techniques.

Trauma-Focused Cognitive Behavioral Therapy (TF-CBT)

Trauma-Focused Cognitive Behavioral Therapy (TF-CBT) is a specialized form of CBT designed to help individuals, particularly children and adolescents, recover from the effects of trauma. TF-CBT is effective in treating PTSD, anxiety, depression, and behavioral problems resulting from traumatic experiences.

Key components of TF-CBT include:

1. **Psychoeducation:** Providing information about trauma and its

effects to help individuals and their families understand the impact of trauma.

2. **Coping Skills:** Teaching relaxation, mindfulness, and emotion regulation skills to manage distress and improve functioning.

3. **Trauma Narrative:** Encouraging individuals to create a narrative of their traumatic experiences to process and integrate the memories.

4. **Cognitive Restructuring:** Identifying and challenging distorted thoughts related to the trauma and developing more adaptive perspectives.

TF-CBT typically involves 12-16 sessions and includes both individual and family components. It is a structured and evidence-based therapy that can produce significant improvements in trauma-related symptoms and overall well-being.

Veterans and men who have experienced trauma can benefit from TF-CBT's structured approach to processing and integrating traumatic memories. The inclusion of family components can also provide additional support and understanding for loved ones.

Please consult your doctor or physician for further details on any of the following treatments.

Pharmacological Treatments

Antidepressants

Antidepressants are commonly used to treat depression, anxiety, and other mood disorders. They work by altering the levels of neurotransmitters in the brain, such as serotonin, norepinephrine, and dopamine, to improve mood and alleviate symptoms.

Common types of antidepressants include:

1. **Selective Serotonin Reuptake Inhibitors (SSRIs):** Such as fluoxetine (Prozac), sertraline (Zoloft), and escitalopram (Lexapro).

2. **Serotonin-Norepinephrine Reuptake Inhibitors (SNRIs):** Such as venlafaxine (Effexor) and duloxetine (Cymbalta).

3. **Tricyclic Antidepressants (TCAs):** Such as amitriptyline (Elavil) and nortriptyline (Pamelor).

4. **Monoamine Oxidase Inhibitors (MAOIs):** Such as phenelzine (Nardil) and tranylcypromine (Parnate).

Antidepressants can be highly effective in reducing symptoms of depression and anxiety, but they may also have side effects. It is important for individuals to work closely with their healthcare providers to find the most appropriate medication and dosage for their needs.

For men, it is essential to address any concerns about medication adherence and potential side effects. Healthcare providers should provide clear information and support to help men understand the benefits and risks of antidepressants.

Anti-Anxiety Medications

Anti-anxiety medications, also known as anxiolytics, are used to treat anxiety disorders and acute anxiety symptoms. These medications can help reduce excessive worry, panic attacks, and physical symptoms of anxiety.

Common types of anti-anxiety medications include:

1. **Benzodiazepines:** Such as diazepam (Valium), lorazepam (Ativan), and alprazolam (Xanax). Benzodiazepines are effective for short-term relief of anxiety but can be habit-forming and are generally not recommended for long-term use.
2. **Buspirone:** An anxiolytic medication that is used for the long-term treatment of generalized anxiety disorder (GAD) and has a lower risk of dependence compared to benzodiazepines.
3. **Beta-Blockers:** Such as propranolol (Inderal), which are sometimes used to manage physical symptoms of anxiety, such as rapid heartbeat and trembling.

Anti-anxiety medications can be effective in managing anxiety symptoms, but they should be used under the guidance of a healthcare provider to minimize the risk of dependence and side effects.

For veterans and men with high-stress occupations, healthcare providers should carefully consider the potential impact of anti-anxiety medications on daily functioning and safety.

Mood Stabilizers

Mood stabilizers are used to treat mood disorders, such as bipolar disorder, by stabilizing mood swings and preventing episodes of mania and depression.

Common types of mood stabilizers include:

1. **Lithium:** A classic mood stabilizer that is highly effective in preventing manic and depressive episodes in bipolar disorder.
2. **Anticonvulsants:** Such as valproate (Depakote), lamotrigine (Lamictal), and carbamazepine (Tegretol), which are also used as mood stabilizers.
3. **Atypical Antipsychotics:** Such as quetiapine (Seroquel) and olanzapine (Zyprexa), which can be used as adjunctive treatments for mood stabilization.

Mood stabilizers can be highly effective in managing mood disorders, but they may have side effects and require regular monitoring by a healthcare provider.

For men, particularly veterans, who may be managing multiple health conditions, careful monitoring and coordination of care are essential to ensure the safe and effective use of mood stabilizers.

Integrative and Holistic Approaches

Mindfulness and Meditation

Mindfulness and meditation are integrative approaches that can enhance mental health and well-being. These practices involve cultivating present-moment awareness and non-judgmental acceptance of thoughts and feelings.

Benefits of mindfulness and meditation include:

1. **Stress Reduction:** Reducing stress and promoting relaxation.
2. **Emotional Regulation:** Improving the ability to manage emotions and reduce reactivity.
3. **Cognitive Flexibility:** Enhancing cognitive flexibility and reducing rumination.
4. **Overall Well-Being:** Promoting a sense of peace, clarity, and well-being.

Mindfulness-based interventions, such as Mindfulness-Based Stress Reduction (MBSR) and Mindfulness-Based Cognitive Therapy (MBCT), have been shown to be effective in reducing symptoms of depression, anxiety, and PTSD.

For men and veterans, mindfulness and meditation can provide practical tools for managing stress and emotional challenges. These practices can be easily integrated into daily routines and can be particularly beneficial for individuals experiencing high levels of stress.

Yoga and Physical Exercise

Yoga and physical exercise are holistic approaches that can improve mental health through physical movement, breath control, and mindfulness.

Benefits of yoga and physical exercise include:

1. **Stress Reduction:** Reducing stress and promoting relaxation.
2. **Improved Mood:** Enhancing mood and reducing symptoms of depression and anxiety.
3. **Physical Health:** Improving physical health and fitness, which can have positive effects on mental well-being.
4. **Mind-Body Connection:** Strengthening the mind-body connection and promoting overall well-being.

Yoga practices, such as Hatha yoga and Vinyasa yoga, combine physical postures, breath control, and meditation to promote mental and physical health. Regular physical exercise, such as aerobic exercise and strength training, has also been shown to have significant mental health benefits.

For men and veterans, incorporating yoga and physical exercise into their routines can provide a healthy outlet for stress and improve overall well-being. These activities can also foster a sense of community and support when done in group settings.

Nutritional and Lifestyle Changes

Nutritional and lifestyle changes can have a profound impact on mental health. A balanced diet, regular exercise, adequate sleep, and stress management are essential components of a healthy lifestyle that supports mental well-being.

Key components of nutritional and lifestyle changes include:

1. **Healthy Diet:** Consuming a balanced diet rich in fruits, vegetables, whole grains, lean proteins, and healthy fats to support brain health and overall well-being.

2. **Regular Exercise:** Engaging in regular physical activity to improve mood, regular physical activity helps reduce stress and enhance overall health.

3. **Adequate Sleep:** Ensuring sufficient and quality sleep to support mental and physical health. Sleep is crucial for cognitive function, mood regulation, and overall well-being.

4. **Stress Management:** Incorporating stress management techniques, such as mindfulness, relaxation exercises, and hobbies, to reduce stress and improve well-being.

For men and veterans, making informed choices about nutrition and lifestyle can significantly impact their mental health. Simple changes, such as reducing the intake of processed foods and increasing physical activity, can lead to substantial improvements in mood and energy levels.

Healthcare providers can work with individuals to develop personalized plans that incorporate nutritional and lifestyle changes to support mental health and overall wellness. Providing education on the connection between diet, exercise, sleep, and mental health can empower men and veterans to make healthier choices.

Integrating Multiple Approaches

Integrating multiple approaches to mental health treatment can provide a comprehensive and holistic approach to care. Combining traditional therapies, innovative treatments, pharmacological interventions, and integrative approaches can address the unique needs and preferences of individuals.

Key principles of integrative mental health care include:

1. **Personalized Treatment:** Tailoring treatments to meet the specific needs and preferences of each individual. This approach recognizes that there is no one-size-fits-all solution to mental health care.

2. **Collaboration:** Encouraging collaboration between healthcare providers, mental health professionals, and individuals to develop

comprehensive treatment plans. This includes coordinating care among primary care physicians, psychiatrists, therapists, and other specialists.

3. **Holistic Approach:** Addressing physical, mental, and social factors that impact mental health and well-being. This involves considering the whole person, including their physical health, emotional state, social connections, and environmental influences.

4. **Continuity of Care:** Ensuring continuity of care and ongoing support to maintain improvements and prevent relapse. Long-term follow-up and support can help individuals sustain their progress and continue to build resilience.

For men and veterans, an integrative approach can be particularly beneficial in addressing the complex interplay of factors that affect their mental health. This approach can provide a more comprehensive and supportive framework for achieving and maintaining mental well-being.

Case Examples and Applications

Case Example 1: Veteran with PTSD

John is a 35-year-old veteran who served in Iraq and Afghanistan. He has been experiencing symptoms of PTSD, including nightmares, flashbacks, and hypervigilance. John also struggles with depression and has turned to alcohol to cope with his symptoms.

Treatment Plan:

1. **Initial Assessment:** Conduct a thorough assessment to understand John's symptoms, history, and needs.

2. **Trauma-Focused Cognitive Behavioral Therapy (TF-CBT):** Start with TF-CBT to help John process and integrate his traumatic experiences.

3. **Medication Management:** Prescribe an SSRI to help manage John's depression and anxiety symptoms.

4. **Substance Use Counseling:** Provide counseling to address John's alcohol use and develop healthier coping strategies.

5. **Mindfulness and Relaxation Techniques:** Introduce mindfulness

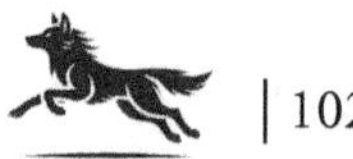

practices and relaxation exercises to help John manage stress and reduce hypervigilance.

6. **Peer Support Group:** Encourage participation in a peer support group for veterans to provide social support and reduce isolation.

Outcome: Over several months, John experiences a reduction in PTSD and depression symptoms. He learns healthier coping strategies, reduces his alcohol use, and builds a supportive network of fellow veterans.

Case Example 2: Male Executive with Anxiety

Michael is a 42-year-old executive who has been experiencing high levels of anxiety due to work-related stress. He struggles with constant worry, difficulty sleeping, and physical symptoms such as tension headaches and palpitations.

Treatment Plan:

1. **Initial Assessment:** Conduct a comprehensive assessment to understand Michael's anxiety symptoms, work environment, and overall health.

2. **Cognitive Behavioral Therapy (CBT):** Start with CBT to help Michael identify and challenge negative thought patterns and develop healthier coping strategies.

3. **Mindfulness-Based Stress Reduction (MBSR):** Introduce MBSR to help Michael manage stress and improve emotional regulation.

4. **Lifestyle Changes:** Recommend changes to Michael's diet, exercise routine, and sleep habits to support overall health and reduce anxiety symptoms.

5. **Pharmacological Intervention:** Consider prescribing a low-dose SSRI or beta-blocker to manage acute anxiety symptoms if necessary.

6. **Workplace Interventions:** Suggest workplace interventions such as flexible scheduling, delegation of tasks, and improved work-life balance.

Outcome: Michael experiences a significant reduction in anxiety symptoms. He learns effective stress management techniques, improves his sleep and overall health, and finds a better balance between work and personal life.

Case Example 3: Adolescent with Depression

James is a 16-year-old high school student who has been struggling with depression. He feels hopeless, has lost interest in activities he once enjoyed, and is experiencing academic difficulties.

Treatment Plan:

1. **Initial Assessment:** Conduct a thorough assessment to understand James's symptoms, history, family dynamics, and academic challenges.
2. **Interpersonal Therapy (IPT):** Start with IPT to address issues related to James's relationships and social interactions.
3. **Cognitive Behavioral Therapy (CBT):** Incorporate CBT to help James develop healthier thought patterns and coping strategies.
4. **Family Therapy:** Include family therapy sessions to improve communication and support within the family.
5. **School Interventions:** Work with school counselors and teachers to provide academic support and accommodations.
6. **Lifestyle Changes:** Encourage regular physical activity, a balanced diet, and adequate sleep to support James's overall health and well-being.

Outcome: James shows improvement in his depression symptoms. He develops healthier relationships, improves his academic performance, and gains a sense of hope and motivation.

A wide range of therapies and treatments are available to address mental health issues, each with its own strengths and benefits. By understanding and utilizing traditional therapies, innovative treatments, pharmacological interventions, and integrative approaches, healthcare providers can offer comprehensive and effective care to individuals experiencing mental health challenges.

The next chapter will explore the cultural factors affecting men's mental health and how different cultures deal with mental health issues, particularly focusing on male mental health.

Chapter 10

Cultural Factors Affecting Men's Mental Health

Introduction to Cultural Factors and Men's Mental Health

Cultural factors play a significant role in shaping men's mental health experiences and behaviors. Understanding the cultural context is essential for effectively addressing mental health issues and promoting well-being among men. This chapter explores how cultural norms, values, and attitudes impact men's mental health, focusing on the differences in cultural approaches and the implications for mental health care. It also examines the specific cultural considerations for veterans and provides insights into how different cultures address mental health challenges, particularly for men.

Cultural Attitudes Towards Mental Health

Overview of Cultural Norms and Values Related to Mental Health

Cultural norms and values significantly influence how mental health is perceived, understood, and addressed. These norms and values shape attitudes towards mental health, including beliefs about the causes of mental health issues, appropriate ways to cope, and the acceptability of seeking help. Different cultures have varying perspectives on mental health, which can impact how individuals experience and respond to mental health challenges.

In many Western cultures, there is a growing recognition of the importance of mental health and a push towards reducing stigma and increasing access to mental health services. However, despite progress, stigma and misconceptions about mental health persist. In contrast, some non-Western cultures may have more traditional views on mental health, often viewing mental health issues as a sign of personal weakness or a result of supernatural forces.

For example, in many Asian cultures, mental health issues are often seen as a source of shame, not only for the individual but also for their family. This can lead to a reluctance to seek help and a preference for addressing mental health issues privately or within the family. Similarly, in many African cultures, mental health problems may be attributed to spiritual or supernatural causes, leading individuals to seek help from traditional healers rather than mental health professionals.

In many Indigenous cultures, mental health is viewed holistically, emphasizing the interconnectedness of physical, mental, emotional, and spiritual well-being. Traditional healing practices and community support are often important aspects of mental health care. However, there may be significant barriers to accessing mainstream mental health services, and stigma and discrimination can impact mental health outcomes.

Differences in Cultural Attitudes Towards Mental Health Across Various Cultures

Different cultures have unique attitudes towards mental health, which can impact how mental health issues are recognized and addressed. Here are some examples of cultural differences in attitudes towards mental health:

1. **Western Cultures:** In many Western cultures, mental health is increasingly recognized as an important aspect of overall health. There is a growing emphasis on reducing stigma, increasing awareness, and providing access to mental health services. However, stigma and misconceptions about mental health still exist, and men may be particularly reluctant to seek help due to cultural expectations of self-reliance and stoicism.

2. **Asian Cultures:** In many Asian cultures, mental health issues are often viewed as a source of shame and a reflection of personal or family failure. This can lead to a reluctance to seek help and a preference for keeping mental health issues private. There may also be a greater emphasis on somatic symptoms, with individuals expressing mental health issues through physical complaints rather than emotional or psychological symptoms.

3. **African Cultures:** In many African cultures, mental health issues may be attributed to spiritual or supernatural causes. This can lead individuals to seek help from traditional healers rather than mental health professionals. Stigma and misconceptions about mental health are also prevalent, and there may be limited access to mental health services.

4. **Latino Cultures:** In many Latino cultures, mental health issues may be viewed as a sign of personal weakness or a result of spiritual or moral failing. There may be a preference for seeking help from family, community, or religious leaders rather than mental health professionals. Stigma and misconceptions about mental health are common, and there may be barriers to accessing mental health services.

5. **Indigenous Cultures:** In many Indigenous cultures, mental health is viewed holistically, with an emphasis on the interconnectedness of physical, mental, emotional, and spiritual well-being. Traditional healing practices and community support are often important aspects of mental health care. However, there may be significant barriers to accessing mainstream mental health services, and stigma and discrimination can impact mental health outcomes.

Impact of Cultural Attitudes on Men's Mental Health

Cultural attitudes towards mental health can significantly impact men's mental health experiences and behaviors. In cultures where mental health issues are stigmatized or viewed as a sign of weakness, men may be particularly reluctant to seek help. This can lead to untreated mental health issues and negative outcomes, such as increased stress, anxiety, depression, and substance use.

Cultural expectations of masculinity can also play a role in how men experience and respond to mental health issues. In many cultures, men are expected to be strong, self-reliant, and stoic, which can make it difficult for them to express vulnerability or seek help for mental health issues. These cultural norms can lead to a reluctance to acknowledge mental health problems and a preference for coping strategies that align with traditional masculine roles, such as suppressing emotions or engaging in risky behaviors.

Understanding the cultural context is essential for effectively addressing men's mental health issues. Culturally sensitive approaches to mental health care can help reduce stigma, encourage help-seeking behaviors, and improve mental health outcomes for men.

Stigma and Help-Seeking Behaviors

Analysis of Stigma Related to Mental Health in Different Cultures

Stigma related to mental health is a significant barrier to seeking help and accessing mental health services. Stigma can manifest in various ways, including negative attitudes and beliefs about mental health, discrimination and exclusion of individuals with mental health issues, and internalized shame and self-stigma.

In many cultures, mental health stigma is rooted in cultural norms and values that view mental health issues as a sign of personal weakness or moral failing. This can lead to negative attitudes and beliefs about mental health and a reluctance to seek help. In some cultures, mental health stigma may also be influenced by spiritual or supernatural beliefs, leading individuals to seek help from traditional healers rather than mental health professionals.

For example, in many Asian cultures, mental health stigma is pervasive, with mental health issues often viewed as a source of shame and a reflection of personal or family failure. This can lead to a reluctance to seek help and a preference for keeping mental health issues private. Similarly, in many African cultures, mental health problems may be attributed to spiritual or supernatural causes, leading individuals to seek help from traditional healers rather than mental health professionals.

How Stigma Affects Men's Willingness to Seek Help

Stigma related to mental health can significantly impact men's willingness to seek help. In cultures where mental health issues are stigmatized, men may be particularly reluctant to seek help due to cultural expectations of masculinity and self-reliance. This can lead to untreated mental health issues and negative outcomes, such as increased stress, anxiety, depression, and substance use.

Cultural expectations of masculinity can also play a role in how men experience and respond to mental health issues. In many cultures, men are expected to be strong, self-reliant, and stoic, which can make it difficult for them to express vulnerability or seek help for mental health issues. These cultural norms can lead to a reluctance to acknowledge mental health problems and a preference for coping strategies that align with traditional masculine roles, such as suppressing emotions or engaging in risky behaviors.

For example, in many Western cultures, men may be reluctant to seek help for mental health issues due to cultural expectations of self-reliance and stoicism. This can lead to untreated mental health issues and negative outcomes, such as increased stress, anxiety, depression, and substance use. Similarly, in many Asian cultures, men may be reluctant to seek help due to cultural norms that view mental health issues as a source of shame and a reflection of personal or family failure.

Strategies for Reducing Stigma and Encouraging Help-Seeking Behaviors

Reducing stigma and encouraging help-seeking behaviors is essential for improving men's mental health outcomes. Here are some strategies for reducing stigma and encouraging help-seeking behaviors:

1. **Public Awareness Campaigns:** Public awareness campaigns can help reduce stigma by increasing understanding and awareness of mental health issues. These campaigns can challenge negative stereotypes and promote positive attitudes towards mental health and help-seeking behaviors.

2. **Education and Training:** Education and training programs for healthcare providers, educators, employers, and community leaders can help reduce stigma and improve understanding of mental health issues. These programs can provide information on the signs and symptoms of mental health issues, effective treatments, and the importance of seeking help.

3. **Peer Support Programs:** Peer support programs can provide a safe and supportive environment for individuals to share their experiences and seek help. Peer support can help reduce stigma and encourage help-seeking behaviors by providing a sense of connection and understanding.

4. **Culturally Sensitive Approaches:** Culturally sensitive approaches to mental health care can help reduce stigma and improve help-seeking behaviors by addressing the unique needs and preferences of different cultural groups. This can include incorporating traditional healing practices, providing services in multiple languages, and involving community leaders in mental health initiatives.

5. **Policy and Advocacy:** Policy and advocacy efforts can help reduce stigma and improve access to mental health services. This can include advocating for policies that promote mental health awareness and education, increase funding for mental health services, and protect the rights of individuals with mental health issues.

6. **Media Representation:** Positive and accurate representation of mental health issues in the media can help reduce stigma and encourage help-seeking behaviors. Media can play a powerful role in shaping public attitudes towards mental health and promoting understanding and acceptance.

Cultural Norms and Masculinity

Exploration of Cultural Norms Related to Masculinity and Their Impact on Men's Mental Health

Cultural norms related to masculinity can significantly impact men's mental health experiences and behaviors. In many cultures, traditional masculine norms emphasize traits such as strength, self-reliance, stoicism, and emotional control. While these traits can be positive, they can also create barriers to seeking help and addressing mental health issues.

For example, traditional masculine norms may discourage men from expressing vulnerability or seeking help for mental health issues. Men may feel pressure to maintain a façade of strength and self-reliance, even when they are struggling. This can lead to untreated mental health issues, increased stress, and negative coping strategies, such as substance use or aggression.

Cultural norms related to masculinity can also impact how men perceive and respond to mental health issues. Men may be more likely to experience mental health issues as physical symptoms, such as headaches, fatigue, or gastrointestinal problems, rather than emotional or psychological symptoms. This can make it difficult for men to recognize and address mental health issues.

How Traditional Masculine Norms Influence Mental Health and Help-Seeking Behaviors

Traditional masculine norms can influence how men experience and respond to mental health issues in several ways:

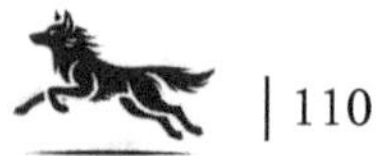

1. **Emotional Suppression:** Traditional masculine norms often discourage men from expressing emotions, particularly vulnerability, sadness, or fear. This can lead to emotional suppression and difficulty recognizing and addressing mental health issues.
2. **Self-Reliance:** Cultural expectations of self-reliance can make it difficult for men to seek help for mental health issues. Men may feel pressure to solve problems on their own and may view seeking help as a sign of weakness.
3. **Stoicism:** Traditional masculine norms often value stoicism and emotional control. Men may feel pressure to maintain a façade of strength and control, even when they are struggling with mental health issues.
4. **Risk-Taking Behavior:** Traditional masculine norms may encourage risk-taking behaviors, such as substance use or aggression, as a way to cope with stress and emotional challenges. These behaviors can exacerbate mental health issues and create additional barriers to seeking help.
5. **Perception of Mental Health Services:** Men may view mental health services as being geared towards women or as incompatible with traditional masculine norms. This can create additional barriers to seeking help and accessing mental health care.

Challenges in Addressing Mental Health Within the Context of Cultural Masculinity Norms

Addressing mental health within the context of cultural masculinity norms presents several challenges:

1. **Stigma and Shame:** Traditional masculine norms can create stigma and shame around mental health issues, making it difficult for men to seek help and access mental health services.
2. **Lack of Awareness:** Men may have limited awareness of mental health issues and the availability of mental health services. This can create barriers to recognizing and addressing mental health issues.
3. **Negative Coping Strategies:** Traditional masculine norms may encourage negative coping strategies, such as substance use or aggression, which can exacerbate mental health issues and create additional barriers to seeking help.

4. **Limited Access to Culturally Sensitive Services:** Men may have limited access to culturally sensitive mental health services that address their unique needs and preferences. This can create barriers to seeking help and accessing mental health care.

5. **Resistance to Change:** Traditional masculine norms can be deeply ingrained and resistant to change. Efforts to address mental health within the context of cultural masculinity norms may require significant cultural shifts and ongoing advocacy and education.

Cultural Considerations for Veterans

Specific Cultural Factors Affecting Veterans' Mental Health

Veterans represent a unique population with distinct cultural factors that impact their mental health. These factors include military culture, experiences of trauma and combat, and the challenges of transitioning to civilian life. Understanding these cultural factors is essential for effectively addressing veterans' mental health issues.

1. **Military Culture:** Military culture emphasizes strength, resilience, and self-reliance. While these traits can be positive, they can also create barriers to seeking help for mental health issues. Veterans may feel pressure to maintain a façade of strength and control, even when they are struggling with mental health issues.

2. **Experiences of Trauma and Combat:** Veterans may have experienced trauma and combat, which can have a significant impact on mental health. These experiences can lead to conditions such as PTSD, depression, and anxiety, and may create additional barriers to seeking help.

3. **Challenges of Transitioning to Civilian Life:** Transitioning from military to civilian life can be challenging and stressful for veterans. This transition can create additional mental health challenges, such as feelings of isolation, loss of identity, and difficulty finding employment.

4. **Stigma and Shame:** Veterans may face stigma and shame related to mental health issues, both within the military and in civilian life. This can create barriers to seeking help and accessing mental health services.

Differences in Cultural Attitudes Towards Veterans and Their Mental Health

Different cultures have unique attitudes towards veterans and their mental health, which can impact how veterans experience and respond to mental health challenges. Here are some examples of cultural differences in attitudes towards veterans and their mental health:

1. **Western Cultures:** In many Western cultures, there is a growing recognition of the mental health challenges faced by veterans and a push towards increasing access to mental health services. However, stigma and misconceptions about mental health still exist, and veterans may be particularly reluctant to seek help due to cultural expectations of strength and resilience.

2. **Asian Cultures:** In many Asian cultures, mental health issues among veterans may be viewed as a source of shame and a reflection of personal or family failure. This can lead to a reluctance to seek help and a preference for keeping mental health issues private.

3. **African Cultures:** In many African cultures, mental health issues among veterans may be attributed to spiritual or supernatural causes. This can lead individuals to seek help from traditional healers rather than mental health professionals.

4. **Latino Cultures:** In many Latino cultures, mental health issues among veterans may be viewed as a sign of personal weakness or a result of spiritual or moral failing. There may be a preference for seeking help from family, community, or religious leaders rather than mental health professionals.

5. **Indigenous Cultures:** In many Indigenous cultures, mental health is viewed holistically, with an emphasis on the interconnectedness of physical, mental, emotional, and spiritual well-being. Traditional healing practices and community support are often important aspects of mental health care for veterans.

Culturally Sensitive Approaches to Supporting Veterans' Mental Health

Culturally sensitive approaches to supporting veterans' mental health are essential for effectively addressing their unique needs and preferences. Here are some strategies for providing culturally sensitive mental health care to veterans:

1. **Incorporating Military Culture:** Incorporating an understanding of military culture into mental health care can help create a supportive and respectful environment for veterans. This can include acknowledging the unique experiences and challenges of military service and using language and approaches that resonate with veterans.

2. **Addressing Trauma and Combat Experiences:** Providing trauma-informed care that acknowledges and addresses the impact of trauma and combat experiences on mental health is essential for supporting veterans. This can include evidence-based treatments for PTSD, such as EMDR and TF-CBT, as well as peer support and trauma-focused group therapy.

3. **Supporting the Transition to Civilian Life:** Providing support for the transition to civilian life can help address the mental health challenges faced by veterans. This can include job training programs, housing assistance, and mental health services that address the unique challenges of transitioning from military to civilian life.

4. **Reducing Stigma and Encouraging Help-Seeking Behaviors:** Reducing stigma and encouraging help-seeking behaviors is essential for improving mental health outcomes for veterans. This can include public awareness campaigns, education and training programs, and peer support programs that provide a safe and supportive environment for veterans to seek help.

5. **Providing Access to Culturally Sensitive Services:** Providing access to culturally sensitive mental health services that address the unique needs and preferences of veterans is essential for improving mental health outcomes. This can include incorporating traditional healing practices, providing services in multiple languages, and involving community leaders in mental health initiatives.

Comparative Analysis of Mental Health Approaches in Different Cultures

Examination of How Different Cultures Address Men's Mental Health Issues

Different cultures have unique approaches to addressing men's mental health issues, which can provide valuable insights and lessons for improving mental health care. Here are some examples of how different cultures address men's mental health issues:

1. **Western Cultures:** In many Western cultures, there is a growing emphasis on reducing stigma and increasing access to mental health services. This includes public awareness campaigns, education and training programs, and peer support programs. There is also a focus on providing evidence-based treatments, such as CBT and DBT, and integrating mental health care into primary care settings.

2. **Asian Cultures:** In many Asian cultures, there is a preference for addressing mental health issues within the family or community. Traditional healing practices, such as acupuncture, herbal medicine, and meditation, are often used in conjunction with or instead of mainstream mental health services. There is also a focus on somatic symptoms and a holistic approach to mental health care.

3. **African Cultures:** In many African cultures, traditional healing practices, such as spiritual healing, herbal medicine, and community support, are important aspects of mental health care. There is a focus on the interconnectedness of physical, mental, and spiritual well-being, and mental health issues are often addressed within the context of the community.

4. **Latino Cultures:** In many Latino cultures, mental health issues are often addressed within the family or community, with a preference for seeking help from family, community, or religious leaders. There is also a focus on traditional healing practices, such as curanderismo, which combines elements of spirituality, herbal medicine, and folk healing.

5. **Indigenous Cultures:** In many Indigenous cultures, mental health is viewed holistically, with an emphasis on the interconnectedness

of physical, mental, emotional, and spiritual well-being. Traditional healing practices, such as sweat lodges, talking circles, and herbal medicine, are important aspects of mental health care. There is also a focus on community support and the importance of cultural identity and connection.

Examples of Effective Mental Health Interventions in Various Cultural Contexts

Effective mental health interventions in various cultural contexts can provide valuable insights and lessons for improving mental health care. Here are some examples of effective mental health interventions in different cultural contexts:

1. **Western Cultures:** In many Western cultures, effective mental health interventions include evidence-based treatments, such as CBT, DBT, and EMDR, as well as public awareness campaigns and peer support programs. Integrating mental health care into primary care settings and providing access to culturally sensitive services have also been effective in improving mental health outcomes.

2. **Asian Cultures:** In many Asian cultures, effective mental health interventions include traditional healing practices, such as acupuncture, herbal medicine, and meditation, as well as family and community support. Integrating traditional healing practices with mainstream mental health services and providing culturally sensitive care have been effective in improving mental health outcomes.

3. **African Cultures:** In many African cultures, effective mental health interventions include traditional healing practices, such as spiritual healing, herbal medicine, and community support, as well as public awareness campaigns and education and training programs. Integrating traditional healing practices with mainstream mental health services and providing culturally sensitive care have been effective in improving mental health outcomes.

4. **Latino Cultures:** In many Latino cultures, effective mental health interventions include traditional healing practices, such as curanderismo, as well as family and community support. Public awareness campaigns, education and training programs, and peer

support programs have also been effective in reducing stigma and encouraging help-seeking behaviors.

5. **Indigenous Cultures:** In many Indigenous cultures, effective mental health interventions include traditional healing practices, such as sweat lodges, talking circles, and herbal medicine, as well as community support and cultural identity and connection. Integrating traditional healing practices with mainstream mental health services and providing culturally sensitive care have been effective in improving mental health outcomes.

Lessons Learned from Different Cultural Approaches to Mental Health Care

Different cultural approaches to mental health care can provide valuable lessons for improving mental health outcomes. Here are some lessons learned from different cultural approaches to mental health care:

1. **Importance of Cultural Sensitivity:** Providing culturally sensitive care that addresses the unique needs and preferences of different cultural groups is essential for improving mental health outcomes. This can include incorporating traditional healing practices, providing services in multiple languages, and involving community leaders in mental health initiatives.

2. **Integrating Traditional and Mainstream Approaches:** Integrating traditional healing practices with mainstream mental health services can be effective in improving mental health outcomes. This can include combining evidence-based treatments with traditional practices, such as acupuncture, herbal medicine, and meditation.

3. **Community Support and Involvement:** Community support and involvement are important aspects of mental health care in many cultures. Providing community-based mental health services and involving community leaders in mental health initiatives can help reduce stigma, encourage help-seeking behaviors, and improve mental health outcomes.

4. **Holistic Approach:** Many cultures view mental health holistically, with an emphasis on the interconnectedness of physical, mental, emotional, and spiritual well-being. Adopting a holistic approach

to mental health care that addresses all aspects of well-being can be effective in improving mental health outcomes.

5. **Reducing Stigma and Encouraging Help-Seeking Behaviors:** Reducing stigma and encouraging help-seeking behaviors are essential for improving mental health outcomes. Public awareness campaigns, education and training programs, and peer support programs can help reduce stigma and encourage help-seeking behaviors.

6. **Tailoring Interventions to Cultural Contexts:** Tailoring mental health interventions to the cultural contexts of individuals can help improve mental health outcomes. This can include considering cultural norms and values, addressing cultural barriers to seeking help, and providing culturally sensitive care.

Cultural factors play a significant role in shaping men's mental health experiences and behaviors. Understanding the cultural context is essential for effectively addressing mental health issues and promoting well-being among men. By providing culturally sensitive care, integrating traditional and mainstream approaches, and reducing stigma and encouraging help-seeking behaviors, healthcare providers can improve mental health outcomes for men from diverse cultural backgrounds.

The next chapter will explore the influence of social media on mental health, examining both the positive and negative impacts of social media use and providing recommendations for managing social media use to promote mental well-being.

Chapter 11

The Influence of Social Media on Men's Mental Health

Introduction to Social Media and Mental Health

The rise of social media has significantly transformed modern life, influencing how people communicate, share information, and form relationships. Social media platforms like Facebook, Instagram, Twitter, and TikTok have become integral parts of daily life for many individuals, including men. While social media offers numerous benefits, it also presents challenges that can impact mental health. This chapter explores the influence of social media on men's mental health, examining both the positive and negative impacts of social media use. It discusses how social media affects self-esteem, body image, and social connections, and how it can contribute to anxiety, depression, and other mental health issues. The chapter also provides recommendations for managing social media use to promote mental well-being.

Positive Impacts of Social Media

Social Connections and Support

One of the primary benefits of social media is its ability to facilitate social connections and provide support. Social media platforms allow individuals to stay connected with friends and family, build new relationships, and join communities based on shared interests. For men, social media can provide a valuable source of social support and connection, particularly for those who may feel isolated or disconnected in their offline lives.

Social media can also provide a platform for men to share their experiences and seek support for mental health issues. Online communities and support groups can offer a safe and supportive environment for men to discuss their struggles, seek advice, and connect with others who have similar experiences.

This can help reduce feelings of isolation and provide a sense of belonging and connection.

For example, online support groups for mental health conditions, such as depression, anxiety, and PTSD, can provide valuable support and resources for men. These groups can offer a sense of community and connection, as well as practical advice and coping strategies for managing mental health issues.

Social media can also bridge geographical distances, enabling men to maintain connections with loved ones who live far away. This can be particularly important for men who have moved for work, military service, or other reasons and may feel isolated from their support networks. Social media can help maintain these connections and provide a sense of continuity and support.

Access to Mental Health Resources and Information

Social media can also provide access to valuable mental health resources and information. Mental health organizations, professionals, and advocates use social media platforms to share information about mental health conditions, treatments, and support services. This can help increase awareness and understanding of mental health issues and provide individuals with the information and resources they need to seek help and support.

For men who may be reluctant to seek help for mental health issues, social media can provide a low-stigma way to access information and resources. Men can learn about mental health conditions, treatment options, and coping strategies from the comfort and privacy of their own homes. This can help reduce barriers to seeking help and encourage men to take the first steps towards addressing their mental health.

For example, mental health organizations such as the National Alliance on Mental Illness (NAMI) and Mental Health America (MHA) use social media platforms to share information about mental health conditions, treatment options, and support services. These organizations also provide online resources, such as informational articles, videos, and webinars, to help individuals learn about and manage their mental health.

Additionally, social media influencers and mental health advocates can play a crucial role in disseminating mental health information and reducing stigma. Influencers who share their personal experiences with mental health can normalize conversations about mental health and encourage their followers to seek help and support.

Opportunities for Self-Expression and Community Building

Social media provides opportunities for self-expression and community building, which can have positive impacts on mental health. Men can use social media platforms to share their thoughts, experiences, and creative works, and to connect with others who share similar interests and passions. This can help foster a sense of identity, purpose, and connection.

For men who may feel constrained by traditional gender norms and expectations, social media can provide a platform for exploring and expressing their authentic selves. Men can connect with communities that challenge traditional masculine norms and offer alternative models of masculinity. This can help reduce feelings of isolation and provide support for men who may feel marginalized or misunderstood.

For example, social media platforms such as Instagram and TikTok have become popular spaces for men to share their creative works, such as photography, music, and writing, and to connect with communities based on shared interests. These platforms can provide a sense of validation and support, as well as opportunities for personal growth and development.

Men can also find support and community in niche online groups that align with their interests and identities. For example, groups focused on mental health, fitness, hobbies, or specific life experiences can provide a sense of belonging and connection, helping to alleviate feelings of loneliness and isolation.

Negative Impacts of Social Media

Impact on Self-Esteem and Body Image

While social media can provide opportunities for self-expression and connection, it can also have negative impacts on self-esteem and body image. Social media platforms often promote unrealistic and idealized images of beauty, success, and happiness, which can create pressure to conform to these standards. For men, this can lead to negative body image, low self-esteem, and dissatisfaction with their appearance and lives.

Exposure to idealized images of muscular and fit bodies on social media can contribute to body dissatisfaction and unhealthy behaviors, such as excessive exercise, restrictive dieting, and the use of performance-enhancing substances. Men may also feel pressure to present a curated and polished image of their lives on social media, leading to feelings of inadequacy and insecurity when their real lives do not match these idealized images.

Research has shown that social media use is associated with increased body dissatisfaction and disordered eating behaviors in men. For example, a study published in the journal *Body Image* found that social media use was associated with higher levels of body dissatisfaction, drive for muscularity, and disordered eating behaviors in men.

Furthermore, the rise of "fitspiration" content—posts and images that promote fitness and healthy lifestyles—can sometimes have the opposite effect, creating unrealistic expectations and promoting unhealthy behaviors. Men may feel pressured to achieve and maintain an idealized body image, leading to negative mental health outcomes.

Cyberbullying and Online Harassment

Cyberbullying and online harassment are significant issues on social media platforms and can have serious negative impacts on mental health. Men, like women, can be targets of cyberbullying and online harassment, which can lead to increased stress, anxiety, depression, and feelings of isolation.

Cyberbullying can take many forms, including mean or hurtful comments, spreading rumors or false information, and sending threatening or abusive messages. For men, cyberbullying can be particularly damaging because it may challenge traditional masculine norms of strength and resilience. Men may feel pressure to downplay or dismiss the impact of cyberbullying, leading to untreated mental health issues and negative outcomes.

Online harassment can also take the form of "doxxing," where an individual's personal information is publicly shared without their consent, or "trolling," where individuals post inflammatory or offensive comments to provoke and upset others. These behaviors can create a hostile and unsafe online environment, leading to increased stress and anxiety for those targeted.

Research has shown that victims of cyberbullying and online harassment are at increased risk of experiencing mental health issues, such as depression, anxiety, and suicidal ideation. For example, a study published in the journal

JAMA Network Open found that victims of cyberbullying were more likely to experience depression and suicidal thoughts compared to those who were not targeted.

Anxiety, Depression, and Addiction

Social media use has been linked to increased levels of anxiety, depression, and addiction. The constant need for validation and approval on social media can create feelings of anxiety and insecurity, particularly when individuals do not receive the positive feedback they seek. The pressure to present a curated and polished image of one's life can also contribute to feelings of inadequacy and low self-esteem.

The "fear of missing out" (FOMO) is another common experience associated with social media use. Seeing others' highlight reels and idealized lives can create a sense of missing out on experiences and opportunities, leading to feelings of loneliness and dissatisfaction. FOMO can contribute to increased social media use, creating a cycle of negative emotions and compulsive behavior.

Social media addiction is a growing concern, with individuals spending excessive amounts of time on social media platforms to the detriment of their mental health and well-being. Social media addiction can lead to sleep disturbances, decreased productivity, and strained relationships. It can also exacerbate mental health issues, such as anxiety and depression, by creating a constant need for validation and comparison.

Research has shown that excessive social media use is associated with higher levels of anxiety, depression, and addiction. For example, a study published in the journal *Computers in Human Behavior* found that excessive social media use was associated with higher levels of anxiety and depression, as well as symptoms of addiction, such as withdrawal and tolerance.

Impact of Social Media on Specific Groups

Adolescents and Young Men

Adolescents and young men are particularly vulnerable to the negative impacts of social media. During adolescence, individuals are developing their identities and self-esteem, and social media can create pressure to conform to idealized images and standards. This can lead to body dissatisfaction, low self-esteem, and mental health issues, such as anxiety and depression.

Adolescents and young men may also be more susceptible to cyberbullying and online harassment, which can have serious negative impacts on their mental health. The anonymity and reach of social media platforms can make it easier for bullies to target and harass individuals, leading to increased stress, anxiety, and feelings of isolation.

For example, a study published in the journal *JAMA Pediatrics* found that social media use was associated with higher levels of anxiety, depression, and cyberbullying victimization among adolescents. The study also found that social media use was associated with lower self-esteem and body dissatisfaction among young men.

Social media can also impact adolescents' sleep patterns, with many staying up late to engage with social media. This can lead to sleep deprivation, which further exacerbates mental health issues, such as anxiety and depression.

Military Veterans and Active-Duty Personnel

Military veterans and active-duty personnel are another group that can be significantly impacted by social media. Social media can provide valuable support and connection for veterans and active-duty personnel, particularly those who may feel isolated or disconnected from their peers. Online support groups and communities can offer a sense of belonging and connection, as well as practical advice and resources for managing mental health issues.

However, social media can also have negative impacts on the mental health of veterans and active-duty personnel. Exposure to traumatic or distressing content on social media can trigger symptoms of PTSD and other mental health issues. Cyberbullying and online harassment can also be a significant issue, leading to increased stress and anxiety.

For example, a study published in the journal *Military Medicine* found that social media use was associated with higher levels of PTSD symptoms among veterans. The study also found that social media use was associated with higher levels of anxiety and depression among active-duty personnel.

Social media can also contribute to the spread of misinformation and harmful content that can negatively impact veterans' mental health. For example, exposure to content that glorifies violence or promotes harmful stereotypes about veterans can exacerbate mental health issues and contribute to feelings of isolation and distress.

Men with Pre-Existing Mental Health Conditions

Men with pre-existing mental health conditions may be particularly vulnerable to the negative impacts of social media. Social media can exacerbate symptoms of anxiety, depression, and other mental health issues, leading to increased stress and negative outcomes.

For example, men with anxiety may feel increased pressure and insecurity from social media, leading to heightened anxiety symptoms. Men with depression may experience feelings of inadequacy and low self-esteem from comparing themselves to others on social media, leading to worsening depression symptoms.

For example, a study published in the journal *Depression and Anxiety* found that social media use was associated with higher levels of anxiety and depression among individuals with pre-existing mental health conditions. The study also found that social media use was associated with higher levels of negative self-perception and rumination among men with depression.

Social media can also create a sense of isolation and disconnection for men with pre-existing mental health conditions. While social media can provide opportunities for connection and support, it can also create a sense of loneliness and inadequacy when individuals compare themselves to others' highlight reels and idealized lives.

Strategies for Healthy Social Media Use

Setting Boundaries and Managing Screen Time

Setting boundaries and managing screen time is essential for maintaining a healthy relationship with social media. Here are some strategies for setting boundaries and managing screen time:

1. **Set Limits:** Set limits on the amount of time spent on social media each day. This can help prevent excessive use and reduce the negative impacts of social media on mental health.

2. **Designate Tech-Free Times:** Designate specific times of the day as tech-free times, such as during meals or before bed. This can help reduce the impact of social media on sleep and overall well-being.

3. **Use Apps and Tools:** Use apps and tools to monitor and manage screen time. Many smartphones have built-in features that allow users to track their screen time and set limits on app usage.

4. **Create a Balanced Routine:** Create a balanced routine that includes time for social media, as well as time for other activities, such as exercise, hobbies, and social interactions. This can help reduce the negative impacts of social media and promote overall well-being.

5. **Take Breaks:** Take regular breaks from social media to disconnect and recharge. This can help reduce the impact of social media on mental health and prevent burnout.

6. **Mindful Usage:** Practice mindful usage of social media by being aware of how it affects your mood and mental health. If certain activities or interactions on social media are causing stress or anxiety, take steps to address them, such as unfollowing negative accounts or limiting time spent on the platform.

Curating Positive Content and Interactions

Curating positive content and interactions on social media can help create a healthier and more supportive online environment. Here are some strategies for curating positive content and interactions:

1. **Follow Positive Accounts:** Follow accounts that promote positive and supportive content, such as mental health organizations, inspirational figures, and supportive communities. This can help create a more positive and uplifting social media experience.

2. **Engage in Positive Interactions:** Engage in positive interactions with others on social media, such as liking, commenting, and sharing supportive content. This can help create a sense of community and connection.

3. **Limit Exposure to Negative Content:** Limit exposure to negative or harmful content on social media, such as accounts that promote unrealistic beauty standards or negative behaviors. This can help reduce the negative impacts of social media on self-esteem and mental health.

4. **Use Social Media for Support:** Use social media to seek support and connection, such as joining online support groups or communities. This can help reduce feelings of isolation and provide valuable resources and advice.

5. **Be Authentic:** Share authentic and genuine content that reflects your true self and experiences. This can help create a more supportive and positive online environment and encourage others to do the same.

6. **Report and Block Negative Content:** Take action against negative or harmful content by reporting and blocking accounts that engage in cyberbullying or harassment. This can help create a safer and more supportive online environment.

Seeking Professional Help and Support

Seeking professional help and support is essential for managing the negative impacts of social media on mental health. Here are some strategies for seeking professional help and support:

1. **Talk to a Mental Health Professional:** Talk to a mental health professional, such as a therapist or counselor, to address the negative impacts of social media on mental health. A mental health professional can provide valuable support, advice, and coping strategies.

2. **Join Support Groups:** Join support groups, both online and offline, to connect with others who have similar experiences and seek support. Support groups can provide a sense of community and connection, as well as practical advice and resources.

3. **Access Online Resources:** Access online resources, such as informational articles, videos, and webinars, to learn about the impacts of social media on mental health and strategies for managing social media use.

4. **Practice Self-Care:** Practice self-care to promote overall well-being and reduce the negative impacts of social media on mental health. This can include activities such as exercise, mindfulness, relaxation techniques, and hobbies.

5. **Develop a Support Network:** Develop a support network of friends, family, and mental health professionals who can provide support and encouragement. This can help reduce feelings of isolation and provide valuable resources and advice.

Case Examples and Applications

Case Example 1: Adolescent Struggling with Body Image

Tom is a 17-year-old high school student who spends several hours a day on social media platforms such as Instagram and TikTok. He often compares himself to influencers who promote fitness and body-building content. As a result, Tom has developed body dissatisfaction and is engaging in unhealthy behaviors, such as restrictive dieting and excessive exercise.

Intervention Plan:

1. **Initial Assessment:** Conduct a comprehensive assessment to understand Tom's social media usage, body image concerns, and mental health status.

2. **Education and Awareness:** Provide education about the unrealistic nature of social media content and the importance of a balanced perspective on body image.

3. **Limit Social Media Usage:** Encourage Tom to set limits on his social media usage and take regular breaks from social media.

4. **Curate Positive Content:** Help Tom identify and follow positive and supportive accounts that promote body positivity and healthy behaviors.

5. **Therapeutic Support:** Provide therapeutic support, such as cognitive-behavioral therapy (CBT), to address body image concerns and develop healthier coping strategies.

Outcome: Over several months, Tom experiences a reduction in body dissatisfaction and unhealthy behaviors. He develops a healthier perspective on body image and reduces his social media usage. Tom also builds a support network of friends and family who encourage and support his well-being.

Case Example 2: Veteran Experiencing PTSD Triggers on Social Media

John is a 35-year-old veteran who served in Iraq and Afghanistan. He has been diagnosed with PTSD and finds that certain content on social media, such as news articles and videos related to combat, triggers his PTSD symptoms. John also experiences anxiety and depression related to his PTSD.

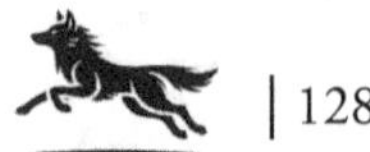

Intervention Plan:
1. **Initial Assessment:** Conduct a comprehensive assessment to understand John's social media usage, PTSD symptoms, and mental health status.
2. **Limit Exposure to Triggers:** Encourage John to limit his exposure to triggering content on social media by using content filters and blocking certain accounts.
3. **Curate Positive Content:** Help John identify and follow positive and supportive accounts that promote mental health and well-being.
4. **Therapeutic Support:** Provide therapeutic support, such as trauma-focused cognitive-behavioral therapy (TF-CBT) and eye movement desensitization and reprocessing (EMDR), to address PTSD symptoms and develop healthier coping strategies.
5. **Peer Support:** Encourage John to join online support groups for veterans to connect with others who have similar experiences and seek support.

Outcome: Over several months, John experiences a reduction in PTSD symptoms and anxiety. He develops healthier coping strategies and reduces his exposure to triggering content on social media. John also builds a support network of fellow veterans who provide encouragement and support.

Case Example 3: Professional Managing Social Media Addiction

Michael is a 42-year-old executive who spends several hours a day on social media platforms for both personal and professional reasons. He finds that his social media usage is affecting his sleep, productivity, and mental health. Michael experiences symptoms of anxiety and depression and feels addicted to social media.

Intervention Plan:
1. **Initial Assessment:** Conduct a comprehensive assessment to understand Michael's social media usage, mental health status, and the impact of social media on his daily life.
2. **Set Limits and Boundaries:** Encourage Michael to set limits on his social media usage and designate tech-free times, such as during meals and before bed.

3. **Use Monitoring Tools:** Recommend the use of apps and tools to monitor and manage screen time.
4. **Therapeutic Support:** Provide therapeutic support, such as cognitive-behavioral therapy (CBT), to address anxiety and depression and develop healthier coping strategies.
5. **Develop a Balanced Routine:** Help Michael develop a balanced routine that includes time for social media, as well as time for other activities, such as exercise, hobbies, and social interactions.

Outcome: Over several months, Michael experiences a reduction in anxiety and depression symptoms and improves his sleep and productivity. He develops a healthier relationship with social media and creates a balanced routine that promotes overall well-being.

Social media has a significant impact on men's mental health, with both positive and negative effects. While social media can provide valuable support, connection, and access to mental health resources, it can also contribute to negative outcomes, such as anxiety, depression, and addiction. By setting boundaries, curating positive content, and seeking professional help and support, men can manage their social media use and promote mental well-being.

The next chapter will highlight specific community programs and initiatives that support men's mental health, with a focus on successful examples and best practices.

Chapter 12

Community Programs and Initiatives Supporting Men's Mental Health

Introduction to Community Programs and Initiatives

Community programs and initiatives play a crucial role in supporting men's mental health by providing valuable resources, reducing stigma, and promoting well-being. These programs offer a variety of services, including counseling, support groups, educational workshops, and outreach activities, to address the unique mental health needs of men. By fostering a sense of community and connection, these initiatives can help men feel supported and empowered to seek help and improve their mental health. This chapter highlights specific community programs and initiatives that support men's mental health, with a focus on successful examples and best practices.

Successful Community Programs and Initiatives

Examples of Effective Community Programs and Initiatives

1. **MENtality Matters (USA):** a non-profit charity based in New York, focused on creating a safe space for all men to be able to reconnect with their true essence, rediscover their strength, purpose, and brotherhood through online community support as well as in-person events throughout the United States of America. They are dedicated to supporting those men who are currently active US military personnel, veterans, and first responders alike. Through transformative retreats, engaging team-building events, and a thriving online community, MENtality Matters provides essential support and fosters a sense of camaraderie and brotherhood among those who have served.

2. **Headspace (Australia):** Headspace is a national youth mental health foundation in Australia that provides early intervention

mental health services to young people aged 12-25. It offers a range of services, including mental health counseling, physical health care, vocational support, and alcohol and drug services. Headspace centers are designed to be youth-friendly and accessible, making it easier for young men to seek help.

3. **Movember Foundation:** The Movember Foundation is a global charity dedicated to improving men's health, particularly mental health and suicide prevention. The foundation raises awareness and funds through its annual Movember campaign, where men grow mustaches during November. The funds support a variety of programs, including mental health initiatives, prostate cancer research, and testicular cancer awareness.

4. **Man Therapy (USA):** Man Therapy is an innovative mental health campaign designed to reach men who may be reluctant to seek help. The campaign uses humor and a fictional character, Dr. Rich Mahogany, to engage men in conversations about mental health. The Man Therapy website offers resources, self-assessments, and information on mental health conditions and treatment options.

5. **The Men's Shed (Ireland, Australia, UK):** The Men's Shed movement is a community-based initiative that provides men with a space to work on projects, socialize, and support each other. Men's Sheds offer a variety of activities, including woodworking, gardening, and community projects, and promote mental well-being by fostering social connections and reducing isolation.

6. **Veterans' Transition Network (Canada):** The Veterans' Transition Network (VTN) is a non-profit organization that provides mental health support and transition services to Canadian veterans. The program offers group-based workshops and peer support to help veterans navigate the challenges of transitioning to civilian life and address mental health issues such as PTSD and depression.

Case Studies of Successful Programs

1. **Headspace (Australia):** Since its inception in 2006, Headspace has grown to include over 100 centers across Australia. The program's youth-friendly approach and comprehensive services have been effective in engaging young men and improving mental health

outcomes. Research has shown that Headspace clients experience significant reductions in psychological distress and improvements in overall well-being.

2. **Movember Foundation:** The Movember Foundation has raised over $1 billion since its founding in 2003, funding over 1,250 men's health projects worldwide. The foundation's focus on mental health and suicide prevention has led to the development of innovative programs and partnerships, such as the "Making Connections" initiative, which aims to create community-based mental health programs for men and boys.

3. **Man Therapy (USA):** Man Therapy has reached millions of men through its humorous and engaging approach to mental health. The campaign's website has received over 1 million visitors, and research has shown that Man Therapy increases men's willingness to seek help and improves their understanding of mental health issues.

4. **The Men's Shed (Ireland, Australia, UK):** The Men's Shed movement has grown rapidly, with thousands of sheds established worldwide. Research has shown that Men's Sheds provide significant mental health benefits, including reduced loneliness, increased social connections, and improved self-esteem. The movement has been particularly effective in reaching older men who may be at risk of social isolation.

5. **Veterans' Transition Network (Canada):** The VTN's group-based workshops and peer support model have been effective in helping veterans navigate the challenges of transitioning to civilian life. Research has shown that participants in VTN programs experience significant improvements in mental health, including reductions in PTSD symptoms and depression.

6. **MENtality Matters (USA):** a non-profit charity based in New York, focused on creating a safe space for all men to be able to reconnect with their true essence, rediscover their strength, purpose, and brotherhood through online community support as well as in-person events throughout the United States of America. They are dedicated to supporting those men who are currently active US military personnel, veterans, and first responders alike. Through transformative retreats, engaging team-building events, and a

thriving online community, MENtality Matters has provided men with a safe space to openly discuss their issues, without stigma or discrimination.

Best Practices for Implementing and Sustaining Community Programs

1. **Community Engagement:** Engaging the community in the development and implementation of mental health programs is essential for ensuring that programs are relevant and effective. This can include involving community members in planning and decision-making processes, conducting needs assessments, and soliciting feedback from program participants.

2. **Cultural Sensitivity:** Providing culturally sensitive care that addresses the unique needs and preferences of different cultural groups is essential for improving mental health outcomes. This can include incorporating traditional healing practices, providing services in multiple languages, and involving community leaders in mental health initiatives.

3. **Collaborative Partnerships:** Building collaborative partnerships with other organizations, such as healthcare providers, schools, and community organizations, can help expand the reach and impact of mental health programs. Partnerships can also provide valuable resources, expertise, and support.

4. **Sustainability Planning:** Developing a sustainability plan that includes funding strategies, program evaluation, and ongoing community engagement is essential for ensuring the long-term success of mental health programs. This can include seeking grants and donations, conducting regular program evaluations, and involving the community in program planning and decision-making.

5. **Evaluation and Adaptation:** Regularly evaluating mental health programs and adapting them based on feedback and outcomes is essential for ensuring their effectiveness. This can include conducting surveys and focus groups, tracking program outcomes, and making data-driven decisions to improve program quality and impact.

Role of Community Organizations

Importance of Community Organizations in Promoting Men's Mental Health

Community organizations play a crucial role in promoting men's mental health by providing accessible and supportive services, reducing stigma, and fostering social connections. These organizations are often deeply rooted in the communities they serve, making them well-positioned to address the unique mental health needs of men.

Community organizations can offer a variety of services, including mental health counseling, support groups, educational workshops, and outreach activities. By providing a safe and supportive environment, these organizations can help men feel more comfortable seeking help and discussing their mental health.

Examples of Community Organizations Supporting Men's Mental Health

1. **MENtality Matters (USA):** a Non-profit charity based in New York, focused on creating a safe space for all men to be able to reconnect with their true essence, rediscover their strength, purpose, and brotherhood through online community support as well as in-person events throughout the United States of America. They are dedicated to supporting those men who are currently active US military personnel, Veterans, and first responders alike. Through transformative retreats, engaging team-building events, and a thriving online community, MENtality Matters provides essential support and fosters a sense of camaraderie and brotherhood among those who have served.

2. **The Samaritans (UK):** The Samaritans is a UK-based charity that provides emotional support to individuals in distress, including men experiencing mental health issues. The organization offers a 24/7 helpline, email support, and face-to-face meetings, providing a confidential and non-judgmental space for individuals to discuss their concerns.

3. **Big White Wall (USA, UK, Australia, New Zealand):** Big White Wall is an online mental health community that provides anonymous support and resources for individuals experiencing mental health issues. The platform offers peer support, self-help resources, and professional counseling, providing a safe and supportive environment for men to seek help.

4. **The Jed Foundation (USA):** The Jed Foundation is a non-profit organization that focuses on promoting mental health and preventing suicide among young adults. The organization works with high schools and colleges to develop mental health programs and resources, providing support and education for young men.

5. **Beyond Blue (Australia):** Beyond Blue is an Australian non-profit organization that provides support and resources for individuals experiencing depression and anxiety. The organization offers a helpline, online chat, and email support, as well as a range of educational resources and community programs.

6. **Mental Health Foundation (New Zealand):** The Mental Health Foundation of New Zealand provides support, resources, and advocacy for individuals experiencing mental health issues. The organization offers a helpline, educational workshops, and community programs, promoting mental health and well-being for men and boys.

Strategies for Community Organizations to Effectively Support Men's Mental Health

1. **Provide Accessible Services:** Ensuring that mental health services are accessible to all members of the community is essential for promoting men's mental health. This can include offering services in multiple languages, providing transportation assistance, and offering flexible appointment times.

2. **Reduce Stigma:** Reducing stigma around mental health is essential for encouraging men to seek help. Community organizations can reduce stigma by providing education and awareness programs, promoting positive attitudes towards mental health, and offering confidential and non-judgmental services.

3. **Foster Social Connections:** Providing opportunities for men to connect with others and build social support networks is essential for promoting mental health. Community organizations can offer support groups, social activities, and community events to foster social connections and reduce isolation.

4. **Involve Men in Program Development:** Involving men in the development and implementation of mental health programs can help ensure that programs are relevant and effective. This can include conducting needs assessments, soliciting feedback, and involving men in planning and decision-making processes.

5. **Provide Culturally Sensitive Care:** Providing culturally sensitive care that addresses the unique needs and preferences of different cultural groups is essential for improving mental health outcomes. This can include incorporating traditional healing practices, providing services in multiple languages, and involving community leaders in mental health initiatives.

Peer Support Groups

Benefits of Peer Support Groups for Men's Mental Health

Peer support groups provide a valuable source of support and connection for men experiencing mental health issues. These groups offer a safe and supportive environment where men can share their experiences, seek advice, and connect with others who have similar experiences. Peer support groups can help reduce feelings of isolation, provide practical advice and resources, and promote mental well-being.

Research has shown that peer support groups can have significant mental health benefits, including reduced symptoms of depression and anxiety, increased social support, and improved self-esteem. Peer support groups can also provide a sense of empowerment and agency, as men take an active role in their mental health and support each other in their recovery.

Examples of Successful Peer Support Groups

1. **Alcoholics Anonymous (AA):** Alcoholics Anonymous is a global peer support group for individuals recovering from alcohol

addiction. The organization offers regular meetings, a 12-step program, and a supportive community, providing a valuable source of support for men experiencing addiction and mental health issues.

2. **Men's Mental Health Support Groups (Various):** Many communities offer men's mental health support groups that provide a safe and supportive environment for men to discuss their mental health issues. These groups often focus on specific issues, such as depression, anxiety, or PTSD, and provide peer support, practical advice, and resources.

3. **Veterans' Peer Support Groups (Various):** Veterans' peer support groups provide a valuable source of support for veterans experiencing mental health issues. These groups offer a safe and supportive environment for veterans to share their experiences, seek advice, and connect with others who have similar experiences.

4. **Online Peer Support Groups (Various):** Online peer support groups provide a valuable source of support and connection for men who may be unable to attend in-person meetings. These groups offer a safe and anonymous space for men to discuss their mental health issues, seek advice, and connect with others who have similar experiences.

Best Practices for Creating and Maintaining Peer Support Groups

1. **Create a Safe and Supportive Environment:** Creating a safe and supportive environment is essential for the success of peer support groups. This can include establishing ground rules, promoting confidentiality, and fostering a non-judgmental and supportive atmosphere.

2. **Provide Training and Support:** Providing training and support for peer support group facilitators is essential for ensuring the success of the group. This can include training on group facilitation, mental health issues, and crisis intervention, as well as ongoing supervision and support.

3. **Promote Accessibility and Inclusivity:** Ensuring that peer support groups are accessible and inclusive is essential for promoting mental health. This can include offering groups in multiple languages,

providing transportation assistance, and promoting inclusivity and diversity within the group.

4. **Encourage Participation and Engagement:** Encouraging participation and engagement within the group is essential for promoting mental health and well-being. This can include fostering a sense of community and connection, promoting active listening and empathy, and providing opportunities for members to take on leadership roles within the group.

5. **Evaluate and Adapt:** Regularly evaluating and adapting peer support groups based on feedback and outcomes is essential for ensuring their effectiveness. This can include conducting surveys and focus groups, tracking group outcomes, and making data-driven decisions to improve group quality and impact.

Innovative Approaches and Programs

Innovative Approaches to Supporting Men's Mental Health

Innovative approaches to supporting men's mental health can provide valuable insights and lessons for improving mental health outcomes. These approaches often involve new and creative ways of addressing mental health issues, reducing stigma, and promoting well-being. Here are some examples of innovative approaches to supporting men's mental health:

1. **Digital Mental Health Platforms:** Digital mental health platforms, such as apps and online therapy services, provide accessible and convenient mental health support for men. These platforms offer a range of services, including therapy, self-help resources, and peer support, and can help reduce barriers to seeking help.

2. **Social Media Campaigns:** Social media campaigns that use humor and relatable content can effectively engage men in conversations about mental health. These campaigns can raise awareness, reduce stigma, and provide valuable resources and support.

3. **Adventure Therapy:** Adventure therapy programs that involve outdoor activities, such as hiking, camping, and rock climbing, can provide a unique and effective way to support men's mental health. These programs promote physical activity, social connection, and personal growth, and can help men build resilience and coping skills.

4. **Workplace Mental Health Programs:** Workplace mental health programs that provide support and resources for employees can help promote mental health and well-being. These programs can include mental health training, employee assistance programs, and workplace wellness initiatives.

Examples of Innovative Programs and Initiatives

1. **BetterHelp:** BetterHelp is an online therapy platform that provides accessible and convenient mental health support. The platform offers therapy sessions with licensed therapists via video, phone, and chat, providing a flexible and confidential way for men to seek help.

2. **The Black Dog Institute (Australia):** The Black Dog Institute is an Australian mental health organization that uses innovative approaches to support mental health. The organization offers digital mental health programs, such as online therapy and self-help resources, as well as research and education programs.

3. **Movember Conversations:** Movember Conversations is an online tool developed by the Movember Foundation that provides practical advice and resources for having conversations about mental health. The tool uses interactive scenarios and relatable content to help men navigate difficult conversations and support their mental health.

4. **Outward Bound Veterans (USA):** Outward Bound Veterans is an adventure therapy program that provides outdoor experiences for veterans to support their mental health and well-being. The program offers a range of activities, including hiking, camping, and rock climbing, and promotes personal growth, resilience, and social connection.

5. **Heads Up Guys (Canada):** Heads Up Guys is a Canadian online resource that provides support and resources for men experiencing depression. The website offers practical advice, self-help resources, and stories from men who have experienced depression, promoting mental health and well-being.

Impact of Innovative Approaches on Men's Mental Health

Innovative approaches to supporting men's mental health can have a significant impact on mental health outcomes. By providing new and creative ways of addressing mental health issues, reducing stigma, and promoting well-being, these approaches can help men feel more comfortable seeking help and improve their mental health.

Research has shown that digital mental health platforms, social media campaigns, and adventure therapy programs can be effective in promoting mental health and well-being. These approaches can help reduce barriers to seeking help, provide practical resources and support, and promote resilience and coping skills.

For example, research on digital mental health platforms has shown that these platforms can effectively reduce symptoms of depression and anxiety and improve overall well-being. Social media campaigns that use humor and relatable content have been shown to increase men's willingness to seek help and improve their understanding of mental health issues. Adventure therapy programs have been shown to promote physical activity, social connection, and personal growth, and can help men build resilience and coping skills.

Community programs and initiatives play a crucial role in supporting men's mental health by providing valuable resources, reducing stigma, and promoting well-being. By implementing successful programs, involving community organizations, creating peer support groups, and using innovative approaches, we can improve mental health outcomes for men. The next chapter will explore practical solutions and recommendations for improving mental health care for men and veterans, highlighting effective strategies and best practices.

Chapter 13

Practical Solutions and Recommendations for Improving Mental Health Care for Men and Veterans

Introduction to Practical Solutions and Recommendations

Improving mental health care for men and veterans is essential for addressing the unique challenges they face and promoting overall well-being. This chapter provides practical solutions and recommendations for enhancing mental health services, reducing stigma, and promoting help-seeking behaviors. It also discusses policy changes, community-based approaches, and innovative programs that can support mental health care for men and veterans.

Enhancing Mental Health Services

Expanding Access to Mental Health Care

Access to mental health care is a critical factor in promoting mental well-being for men and veterans. Expanding access to mental health services involves increasing the availability of mental health providers, reducing financial barriers, and ensuring that services are accessible to all individuals, regardless of their location or socioeconomic status.

1. **Increasing the Availability of Mental Health Providers:**
   - **Educational Initiatives**: Increasing the number of training programs for mental health professionals and providing scholarships or loan forgiveness for those who choose to work in underserved areas.
   - **Recruitment Campaigns**: Launching campaigns to attract professionals to the mental health field, emphasizing the impact and importance of their work.

2. **Reducing Financial Barriers:**
    - **Insurance Coverage**: Advocating for policies that require insurance companies to cover mental health services at the same level as physical health services.
    - **Subsidies and Grants**: Providing subsidies for low-income individuals and grants for community organizations offering mental health services.
3. **Ensuring Geographic Accessibility:**
    - **Telehealth Services**: Expanding the use of telehealth to reach individuals in rural or underserved areas, ensuring they have access to mental health care.
    - **Mobile Clinics**: Implementing mobile mental health clinics that can travel to remote locations, providing services directly to those in need.

Integrating Mental Health Services into Primary Care

Integrating mental health services into primary care can help ensure that men and veterans receive comprehensive and coordinated care. Primary care providers are often the first point of contact for individuals seeking health care, making them well-positioned to identify and address mental health issues.

1. **Training Primary Care Providers:**
    - **Workshops and Seminars**: Offering regular workshops and seminars on mental health for primary care providers to enhance their skills in recognizing and treating mental health conditions.
    - **Certification Programs**: Developing certification programs for primary care providers in mental health care.
2. **Collaborative Care Models:**
    - **Integrated Teams:** Creating integrated care teams that include primary care providers, mental health professionals, and social workers who collaborate on patient care.
    - **Co-Location of Services:** Co-locating mental health services within primary care settings to facilitate easier referrals and more coordinated care.
3. **Screening and Early Intervention:**

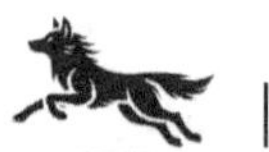

- **Routine Screenings**: Implementing routine mental health screenings for all patients during primary care visits using standardized tools.
- **Early Intervention Programs**: Developing programs that provide immediate support and follow-up care for individuals identified with mental health issues during screenings.

Providing Culturally Sensitive Care

Providing culturally sensitive care that addresses the unique needs and preferences of different cultural groups is essential for improving mental health outcomes for men and veterans. Culturally sensitive care involves understanding and respecting cultural differences, incorporating traditional healing practices, and providing services in multiple languages.

1. **Cultural Competency Training:**
   - **Ongoing Education**: Requiring ongoing cultural competency education for all mental health providers.
   - **Resource Centers**: Establishing resource centers that provide information and training on cultural competence.
2. **Incorporating Traditional Healing Practices:**
   - **Collaborations with Traditional Healers**: Building partnerships with traditional healers to integrate their practices into mental health care.
   - **Holistic Care Models**: Developing holistic care models that incorporate spiritual, physical, and emotional healing practices.
3. **Providing Services in Multiple Languages:**
   - **Bilingual Providers**: Recruiting and training bilingual mental health providers.
   - **Translation Services**: Providing professional translation services and ensuring all informational materials are available in multiple languages.

Reducing Stigma and Promoting Help-Seeking

Public Awareness Campaigns

Public awareness campaigns can help reduce stigma and promote help-seeking behaviors by increasing understanding and awareness of mental health issues. These campaigns can challenge negative stereotypes, promote positive attitudes towards mental health, and provide information on available resources and support.

1. **Media Campaigns:**
   - **Inclusive Messaging**: Creating media campaigns that feature diverse individuals sharing their mental health journeys to normalize seeking help.
   - **Broad Reach**: Utilizing television, radio, print, and online media to reach a wide audience.
2. **Social Media Campaigns:**
   - **Engaging Content**: Developing engaging content that uses humor, relatable stories, and interactive elements to raise awareness.
   - **Influencers and Ambassadors**: Collaborating with social media influencers and mental health ambassadors to spread positive messages about mental health.
3. **Community Outreach:**
   - **Workshops and Presentations**: Hosting workshops and presentations in community centers, schools, and workplaces to educate the public about mental health.
   - **Information Booths**: Setting up information booths at community events to distribute resources and answer questions about mental health.

Education and Training Programs

Education and training programs can help reduce stigma and promote help-seeking behaviors by providing individuals with the knowledge and skills they need to understand and address mental health issues. These programs can target various audiences, including healthcare providers, educators, employers, and community members.

1. **Mental Health First Aid:**
   - **Comprehensive Training**: Offering comprehensive Mental Health First Aid training programs to teach individuals how to recognize and respond to mental health crises.
   - **Community-Based Programs**: Providing community-based training sessions to increase accessibility.

2. **Professional Development for Healthcare Providers:**
   - **Continuing Education**: Requiring continuing education on mental health for all healthcare providers.
   - **Specialized Training**: Offering specialized training programs for healthcare providers working with specific populations, such as veterans.
3. **Workplace Training Programs:**
   - **Employee Workshops**: Providing mental health workshops for employees to educate them about mental health issues and available resources.
   - **Management Training**: Training managers to recognize signs of mental health issues and support employees in seeking help.

Peer Support and Advocacy

Peer support and advocacy can play a crucial role in reducing stigma and promoting help-seeking behaviors. Peer support involves individuals with lived experience of mental health issues providing support and encouragement to others, while advocacy involves promoting positive attitudes towards mental health and advocating for policy changes.

1. **Peer Support Programs:**
   - **Peer Training**: Providing training for peer support workers to ensure they have the skills and knowledge to support others effectively.
   - **Structured Programs**: Developing structured peer support programs that include regular meetings and activities.
2. **Advocacy Campaigns:**
   - **Public Testimonies**: Encouraging individuals with lived experience to share their stories publicly to reduce stigma and promote understanding.
   - **Policy Advocacy**: Engaging in policy advocacy to promote mental health reforms and improvements.
3. **Involving Individuals with Lived Experience:**
   - **Advisory Boards**: Including individuals with lived experience on advisory boards to inform program development and implementation.

- **Leadership Opportunities**: Providing leadership opportunities for individuals with lived experience to take an active role in advocacy and support efforts.

Policy Changes and Advocacy

Policy Recommendations for Improving Mental Health Care

Policy changes can play a crucial role in improving mental health care for men and veterans. These changes can involve increasing funding for mental health services, improving insurance coverage for mental health care, and implementing policies that promote mental health and well-being.

1. **Increasing Funding for Mental Health Services:**
   - **Government Grants**: Advocating for increased government funding for mental health services through grants and subsidies.
   - **Public-Private Partnerships**: Developing public-private partnerships to fund mental health initiatives.
2. **Improving Insurance Coverage for Mental Health Care:**
   - **Parity Laws**: Implementing and enforcing parity laws that require insurance companies to cover mental health services at the same level as physical health services.
   - **Medicaid Expansion**: Expanding Medicaid coverage to include comprehensive mental health services.
3. **Implementing Policies that Promote Mental Health and Well-Being:**
   - **Workplace Mental Health Policies**: Developing and promoting workplace policies that support mental health, such as flexible work arrangements and employee assistance programs.
   - **Mental Health Education in Schools**: Implementing mental health education programs in schools to promote early intervention and awareness.

Advocacy Efforts and Initiatives

Advocacy efforts and initiatives can help raise awareness of mental health issues, reduce stigma, and promote policy changes. These efforts can involve collaboration with policymakers, stakeholders, and community organizations to advocate for mental health reforms and improvements.

1. **Collaborating with Policymakers and Stakeholders:**
   - **Policy Roundtables**: Organizing roundtable discussions with policymakers, stakeholders, and community members to discuss mental health issues and develop policy recommendations.
   - **Legislative Advocacy**: Engaging in legislative advocacy by meeting with lawmakers, providing testimony at hearings, and submitting policy proposals.
2. **Public Advocacy Campaigns:**
   - **Media Outreach**: Conducting media outreach to raise awareness of mental health issues and promote positive attitudes towards mental health.
   - **Community Events**: Hosting community events to engage the public and promote mental health advocacy efforts.
3. **Grassroots Advocacy:**
   - **Community Mobilization**: Mobilizing community members to advocate for mental health reforms through letter-writing campaigns, petitions, and social media advocacy.
   - **Coalition Building**: Building coalitions of advocacy organizations, community groups, and stakeholders to amplify advocacy efforts and promote policy changes.

Community-Based Approaches

Developing Community Mental Health Programs

Community mental health programs can provide valuable support and resources for men and veterans experiencing mental health issues. These programs can involve a range of services, including counseling, support groups, educational workshops, and outreach activities.

1. **Needs Assessment and Planning:**
   - **Community Surveys**: Conducting community surveys to gather information on the mental health needs and preferences of men and veterans.

- **Focus Groups**: Organizing focus groups with community members to discuss mental health needs and develop program ideas.

2. **Collaborating with Community Organizations:**
   - **Partnership Agreements**: Developing partnership agreements with community organizations to provide comprehensive and coordinated mental health services.
   - **Resource Sharing**: Sharing resources, such as funding, staff, and facilities, with community partners to enhance program delivery.

3. **Providing Culturally Sensitive Services:**
   - **Cultural Consultations**: Conducting cultural consultations with community leaders and cultural experts to ensure programs are culturally appropriate.
   - **Multilingual Services**: Offering mental health services in multiple languages to meet the needs of diverse communities.

Building Partnerships with Community Organizations

Building partnerships with community organizations can help expand the reach and impact of mental health programs. These partnerships can provide valuable resources, expertise, and support, and help ensure that programs are relevant and effective.

1. **Identifying Potential Partners:**
   - **Community Mapping**: Conducting community mapping to identify potential partners, such as healthcare providers, schools, and community organizations.
   - **Outreach and Engagement**: Conducting outreach to potential partners and engaging them in discussions about collaboration opportunities.

2. **Developing Collaborative Agreements:**
   - **Memoranda of Understanding (MOUs)**: Developing MOUs that outline the roles, responsibilities, and goals of each partner.
   - **Joint Planning Committees**: Establishing joint planning committees with representatives from each partner organization to oversee program development and implementation.

3. **Providing Training and Support:**
   - **Capacity Building**: Offering capacity-building training for community partners to enhance their ability to deliver effective mental health services.
   - **Technical Assistance**: Providing technical assistance and support to community partners to address challenges and improve program quality.

Involving Men and Veterans in Program Development

Involving men and veterans in the development and implementation of mental health programs can help ensure that programs are relevant and effective. This can involve conducting needs assessments, soliciting feedback, and involving men and veterans in planning and decision-making processes.

1. **Conducting Needs Assessments:**
   - **Surveys and Interviews**: Conducting surveys and interviews with men and veterans to gather information on their mental health needs and preferences.
   - **Community Forums**: Organizing community forums to discuss mental health needs and gather input from men and veterans.
2. **Soliciting Feedback:**
   - **Feedback Mechanisms**: Establishing feedback mechanisms, such as suggestion boxes and online surveys, to gather feedback on program design and implementation.
   - **Focus Groups**: Conducting focus groups with men and veterans to gather detailed feedback on program experiences and suggestions for improvement.
3. **Involving Men and Veterans in Planning and Decision-Making:**
   - **Advisory Committees**: Establishing advisory committees with men and veterans to provide input on program development and implementation.
   - **Participatory Planning**: Involving men and veterans in participatory planning processes, such as community planning workshops and design charrettes.

Innovative Programs and Interventions

Examples of Innovative Programs and Interventions

Innovative programs and interventions can provide valuable insights and lessons for improving mental health outcomes for men and veterans. These programs often involve new and creative ways of addressing mental health issues, reducing stigma, and promoting well-being.

1. **Digital Mental Health Platforms:**
   - **Teletherapy Services**: Offering teletherapy services that provide convenient and confidential mental health support.
   - **Mental Health Apps**: Developing mental health apps that offer self-help resources, mood tracking, and peer support.

2. **Social Media Campaigns:**
   - **Interactive Campaigns**: Creating interactive social media campaigns that engage users through quizzes, polls, and live chats.
   - **Influencer Partnerships**: Partnering with social media influencers to reach a broader audience and promote positive messages about mental health.

3. **Adventure Therapy:**
   - **Outdoor Programs**: Developing outdoor programs that offer adventure therapy activities, such as hiking, camping, and rock climbing, to promote mental health and well-being.
   - **Wilderness Retreats**: Organizing wilderness retreats that provide a supportive environment for men and veterans to connect with nature and each other.

4. **Workplace Mental Health Programs:**
   - **Employee Assistance Programs (EAPs)**: Offering EAPs that provide confidential counseling and support services for employees.
   - **Workplace Wellness Initiatives**: Implementing workplace wellness initiatives that promote physical activity, stress management, and work-life balance.

Evaluating and Scaling Successful Programs

Evaluating and scaling successful programs can help ensure that innovative approaches to supporting men's mental health are effective and sustainable. This can involve conducting program evaluations, identifying best practices, and developing strategies for scaling successful programs.

1. **Conducting Program Evaluations:**
   - **Mixed-Methods Evaluation**: Using mixed-methods evaluation approaches that combine quantitative and qualitative data to assess program outcomes and impact.
   - **Continuous Improvement**: Implementing continuous improvement processes that use evaluation findings to make data-driven decisions and enhance program quality.

2. **Identifying Best Practices:**
   - **Literature Reviews**: Conducting literature reviews to identify best practices and evidence-based approaches in mental health care.
   - **Stakeholder Consultations**: Consulting with stakeholders, including program participants, providers, and community partners, to identify best practices and lessons learned.

3. **Developing Strategies for Scaling Successful Programs:**
   - **Replication Guides**: Developing replication guides that provide detailed instructions and resources for scaling successful programs.
   - **Training and Support**: Providing training and support for new program sites to ensure successful replication and implementation.
   - **Funding and Resources**: Seeking funding and resources to support the expansion of successful programs, including grants, donations, and public-private partnerships.

Improving mental health care for men and veterans requires a comprehensive and multifaceted approach that includes enhancing mental health services, reducing stigma, promoting help-seeking behaviors, and implementing policy changes. By adopting community-based approaches, involving men and veterans in program development, and utilizing innovative programs and interventions, we can improve mental health outcomes and promote well-being for men and veterans.

The next chapter will provide an analysis of current policies and propose changes to further support men's mental health and veterans' mental health care.

Chapter 14

Expert Opinions and Future Directions in Men's and Veterans' Mental Health Care

Introduction to Expert Opinions and Future Directions

Expert insights play a critical role in shaping the future of mental health care for men and veterans. By understanding current trends, challenges, and emerging research, mental health professionals can develop more effective interventions and advocate for necessary policy changes. This chapter provides expert opinions on effective interventions, policy changes, and future directions in men's and veterans' mental health care. It also outlines recommendations for advancing mental health care, emphasizing the importance of innovation, collaboration, and continued advocacy.

Current Trends and Challenges in Men's and Veterans' Mental Health

Overview of Current Mental Health Trends Among Men and Veterans

Mental health trends among men and veterans reveal significant challenges and areas for improvement. Understanding these trends is essential for developing effective interventions and policies.

1. **Rising Rates of Anxiety and Depression:** Recent studies indicate that anxiety and depression rates among men and veterans are increasing. Factors such as economic instability, social isolation, and trauma contribute to these rising rates. For example, a 2021 study published in *JAMA Network Open* found a significant increase in anxiety and depression symptoms among men during the COVID-19 pandemic.

2. **High Suicide Rates:** Suicide rates among men, particularly veterans, remain alarmingly high. The Veterans Affairs' 2020 National Veteran Suicide Prevention Annual Report highlights that veterans are 1.5 times more likely to die by suicide than non-veteran

adults. Experts call for comprehensive suicide prevention strategies, including crisis intervention and ongoing support.

3. **Impact of COVID-19:** The COVID-19 pandemic has exacerbated mental health issues among men and veterans. Increased stress, isolation, and economic uncertainty have led to a surge in mental health problems. According to the American Psychological Association, the pandemic has created a "mental health tsunami" that requires immediate and long-term attention.

4. **Stigma and Barriers to Care:** Stigma and barriers to accessing mental health care persist, preventing many men and veterans from seeking help. Cultural attitudes, financial constraints, and lack of awareness contribute to these barriers. A 2019 report from the National Academies of Sciences, Engineering, and Medicine emphasizes the need for targeted efforts to reduce stigma and improve access to care.

Challenges in Providing Effective Mental Health Care

Providing effective mental health care for men and veterans involves addressing various challenges. Experts identify key areas that require attention to improve mental health outcomes.

1. **Limited Access to Mental Health Services:** Access to mental health services is often limited, particularly in rural and underserved areas. The Health Resources and Services Administration reports that 123 million Americans live in areas with a shortage of mental health professionals. Experts recommend expanding telehealth services and increasing the availability of mental health providers to address this issue.

2. **Insufficient Funding and Resources:** Mental health programs frequently face funding and resource constraints. A 2018 survey by the National Council for Behavioral Health found that 77% of counties in the U.S. reported a shortage of mental health providers. Experts emphasize the need for increased investment in mental health services, including funding for community-based programs and innovative interventions.

3. **Fragmented Care Systems:** The fragmentation of mental health care systems can hinder the delivery of comprehensive

and coordinated care. The Substance Abuse and Mental Health Services Administration (SAMHSA) highlights the importance of integrating mental health, primary care, and social services. Experts advocate for integrated care models that bring together these services to provide holistic care.

4. **Cultural Competency:** Providing culturally competent care is essential for addressing the diverse needs of men and veterans. A 2020 study in the *Journal of Racial and Ethnic Health Disparities* found that cultural competency training for mental health providers improves patient satisfaction and treatment outcomes. Experts highlight the importance of cultural competency training and the integration of culturally relevant practices into care.

Effective Interventions and Best Practices

Expert Opinions on Effective Interventions for Men's and Veterans' Mental Health

Experts in the field of men's and veterans' mental health offer valuable insights into effective interventions. These interventions address various aspects of mental health, from prevention to treatment.

1. **Cognitive-Behavioral Therapy (CBT):** CBT is widely regarded as an effective treatment for anxiety, depression, and PTSD. A meta-analysis published in *Psychological Medicine* in 2020 found that CBT significantly reduces symptoms of depression and anxiety. Experts highlight the success of CBT in helping men and veterans manage their symptoms and improve their mental health.

2. **Peer Support Programs:** Peer support programs provide men and veterans with opportunities to connect with others who share similar experiences. A 2019 study in the *Journal of Military, Veteran and Family Health* found that peer support programs reduce isolation and increase engagement in treatment. Experts emphasize the benefits of peer support in promoting recovery.

3. **Trauma-Informed Care:** Trauma-informed care is crucial for addressing the mental health needs of veterans. A 2020 review in *Trauma, Violence, & Abuse* highlights the effectiveness of trauma-informed practices in improving mental health outcomes. Experts

recommend incorporating trauma-informed practices into all aspects of mental health care, from assessment to treatment.

4. **Mindfulness and Stress Reduction Techniques:** Mindfulness and stress reduction techniques, such as meditation and yoga, have shown promise in improving mental health. A 2018 study in *Mindfulness* found that mindfulness-based interventions reduce symptoms of anxiety and depression. Experts advocate for integrating these practices into mental health programs for men and veterans.

Case Studies and Examples of Successful Programs

1. **Veterans Crisis Line:** The Veterans Crisis Line provides confidential support to veterans in crisis. The program has been successful in preventing suicides and connecting veterans with mental health resources. A 2019 evaluation by the VA found that the Veterans Crisis Line significantly reduces suicidal ideation and distress among callers. Experts highlight the importance of crisis intervention services in addressing urgent mental health needs.

2. **Man Therapy:** Man Therapy is a mental health initiative that uses humor and relatable content to engage men in conversations about mental health. The program has successfully reduced stigma and encouraged help-seeking behaviors among men. A 2018 evaluation by the University of Colorado found that Man Therapy increased men's willingness to seek help and improved mental health outcomes. Experts recommend using creative approaches to engage men in mental health care.

3. **Veterans Integration to Academic Leadership (VITAL):** The VITAL program helps veterans transition to academic life by providing mental health support and resources. The program has improved mental health outcomes and academic success for veterans. A 2019 study in *Psychological Services* found that VITAL participants reported reduced symptoms of PTSD and depression. Experts emphasize the importance of support programs for veterans in educational settings.

4. **Headstrong Project:** The Headstrong Project provides free, confidential mental health care to veterans. The program uses

evidence-based treatments, such as CBT and EMDR, to address PTSD and other mental health issues. A 2020 evaluation by Columbia University found that Headstrong participants experienced significant reductions in PTSD and depression symptoms. Experts highlight the success of the Headstrong Project in providing accessible and effective care to veterans.

Analysis of Best Practices in Mental Health Care

Experts identify several best practices in mental health care that can improve outcomes for men and veterans.

1. **Integrated Care Models:** Integrated care models that combine mental health, primary care, and social services provide comprehensive and coordinated care. A 2020 review in *The Lancet Psychiatry* found that integrated care models improve access to care and treatment outcomes. Experts recommend implementing integrated care models to address the diverse needs of men and veterans.

2. **Community-Based Programs:** Community-based programs that provide accessible and culturally relevant services are essential for improving mental health outcomes. A 2018 study in *Community Mental Health Journal* found that community-based programs increase engagement in treatment and reduce symptoms of anxiety and depression. Experts advocate for increasing funding and support for community-based mental health programs.

3. **Telehealth Services:** Telehealth services can expand access to mental health care, particularly in rural and underserved areas. A 2020 study in *JAMA Psychiatry* found that telehealth services are as effective as in-person therapy in treating mental health conditions. Experts recommend leveraging telehealth to provide timely and convenient care to men and veterans.

4. **Cultural Competency Training:** Providing cultural competency training for mental health providers is crucial for delivering effective care. A 2020 review in *The Journal of Nervous and Mental Disease* found that cultural competency training improves provider-patient communication and treatment outcomes. Experts emphasize the importance of understanding and respecting cultural differences in mental health treatment.

Policy Changes and Advocacy Efforts

Expert Recommendations for Policy Changes to Support Men's and Veterans' Mental Health

Policy changes are essential for improving mental health care for men and veterans. Experts provide recommendations for policy changes that can support mental health initiatives and improve access to care.

1. **Increasing Funding for Mental Health Services:** Experts advocate for increased funding for mental health services, including grants for community-based programs and support for innovative interventions. This funding can help address resource constraints and improve access to care. A 2019 report from the National Alliance on Mental Illness (NAMI) highlights the need for sustained investment in mental health services.

2. **Expanding Telehealth Services:** Experts recommend expanding telehealth services to increase access to mental health care. Policy changes that support telehealth infrastructure and reimbursement can facilitate the widespread adoption of telehealth services. A 2020 report from the American Telemedicine Association emphasizes the importance of telehealth in improving access to care.

3. **Implementing Parity Laws:** Ensuring that mental health services are covered at the same level as physical health services is essential. Experts call for the implementation and enforcement of parity laws to reduce financial barriers to mental health care. A 2018 report from the Mental Health Parity and Addiction Equity Coalition highlights the need for stronger enforcement of parity laws.

4. **Promoting Integrated Care Models:** Policy changes that support integrated care models can improve the delivery of comprehensive and coordinated care. Experts recommend policies that facilitate collaboration between mental health, primary care, and social services. A 2020 review in *Health Affairs* emphasizes the benefits of integrated care models for mental health outcomes.

Analysis of Successful Advocacy Efforts and Initiatives

1. **Mental Health Parity and Addiction Equity Act (MHPAEA):** The MHPAEA requires insurance companies to provide equal coverage for mental health and substance use treatment. Advocacy efforts have been successful in promoting the implementation and enforcement of this law. Experts highlight the importance of continued advocacy to ensure compliance with parity laws.

2. **Veterans Health Administration (VHA) Improvements:** Advocacy efforts have led to improvements in the VHA's mental health services, including increased funding and expanded access to care. Experts emphasize the need for ongoing advocacy to address remaining challenges and improve the quality of care.

3. **Public Awareness Campaigns:** Public awareness campaigns, such as Mental Health Awareness Month, have successfully raised awareness about mental health issues and reduced stigma. Experts recommend continuing these campaigns to promote mental health awareness and encourage help-seeking behaviors.

4. **Grassroots Advocacy:** Grassroots advocacy efforts, such as letter-writing campaigns and community events, have been effective in promoting policy changes. Experts highlight the importance of grassroots advocacy in amplifying the voices of individuals and communities affected by mental health issues.

Strategies for Promoting Policy Changes and Improving Mental Health Care

1. **Building Coalitions:** Building coalitions of advocacy organizations, community groups, and stakeholders can amplify advocacy efforts and promote policy changes. Experts recommend forming coalitions to support mental health initiatives and advocate for necessary reforms.

2. **Engaging Policymakers:** Engaging policy makers through meetings, testimony at legislative hearings, and policy briefings can influence policy changes. Experts emphasize the importance of educating policymakers about the needs and challenges of men and veterans' mental health.

3. **Public Awareness Campaigns:** Conducting public awareness campaigns can raise awareness about mental health issues and promote policy changes. Experts recommend using media, social media, and community events to disseminate information and engage the public.

4. **Grassroots Advocacy:** Mobilizing community members to advocate for mental health reforms through letter-writing campaigns, petitions, and social media advocacy can drive policy changes. Experts highlight the importance of grassroots advocacy in creating a groundswell of support for mental health initiatives.

Emerging Research and Innovations

Overview of Emerging Research in Men's and Veterans' Mental Health

Emerging research in men's and veterans' mental health provides valuable insights into new treatment approaches and interventions.

1. **Digital Mental Health Interventions:** Digital mental health interventions, such as mobile apps and online therapy programs, are gaining popularity. Research published in *JMIR Mental Health* in 2020 indicates that these interventions can be effective in improving mental health outcomes and increasing access to care.

2. **Neurobiological Research:** Advances in neurobiological research are shedding light on the underlying mechanisms of mental health conditions. This research can inform the development of targeted treatments and interventions for men and veterans. A 2020 review in *Nature Neuroscience* highlights recent advances in understanding the neurobiology of PTSD and depression.

3. **Psychosocial Interventions:** Emerging research on psychosocial interventions, such as group therapy and peer support programs, highlights their effectiveness in improving mental health outcomes. A 2019 study in *Psychiatric Services* found that psychosocial interventions reduce symptoms of anxiety, depression, and PTSD.

4. **Trauma-Informed Care:** Research on trauma-informed care emphasizes the importance of addressing trauma in mental health treatment. Emerging studies suggest that trauma-informed practices can improve treatment outcomes for men and veterans

with a history of trauma. A 2020 review in *The American Journal of Psychiatry* supports the effectiveness of trauma-informed care in treating PTSD.

Innovative Approaches and Technologies in Mental Health Care

Innovative approaches and technologies are transforming mental health care for men and veterans.

1. **Virtual Reality Therapy:** Virtual reality (VR) therapy is an emerging treatment for PTSD and anxiety. VR therapy immerses individuals in controlled virtual environments to help them process traumatic experiences and reduce symptoms. A 2020 study in *The Lancet Psychiatry* found that VR therapy significantly reduces PTSD symptoms in veterans.

2. **Teletherapy and Telepsychiatry:** Teletherapy and telepsychiatry use video conferencing technology to provide mental health care remotely. These services increase access to care, particularly in rural and underserved areas. A 2020 review in *The Journal of Clinical Psychiatry* found that teletherapy and telepsychiatry are as effective as in-person therapy in treating mental health conditions.

3. **Wearable Devices:** Wearable devices, such as fitness trackers and smartwatches, can monitor physiological indicators of stress and anxiety. These devices can provide real-time feedback and support mental health interventions. A 2019 study in *Journal of Medical Internet Research* found that wearable devices can enhance self-monitoring and improve mental health outcomes.

4. **Artificial Intelligence (AI) and Machine Learning:** AI and machine learning are being used to analyze mental health data and develop personalized treatment plans. These technologies can identify patterns and predict treatment outcomes, improving the effectiveness of mental health care. A 2020 review in *The Lancet Digital Health* highlights the potential of AI and machine learning in enhancing diagnostic accuracy and treatment planning.

Expert Predictions for Future Developments in the Field

Experts predict several future developments in men's and veterans' mental health care.

1. **Personalized Medicine:** Advances in personalized medicine will enable tailored treatment plans based on individual genetic, biological, and psychosocial factors. Experts predict that personalized medicine will improve treatment outcomes and reduce trial-and-error approaches to mental health care. A 2020 review in *Nature Reviews Genetics* highlights the potential of personalized medicine in mental health treatment.

2. **Integration of Technology:** The integration of technology, such as telehealth, VR therapy, and AI, will continue to transform mental health care. Experts anticipate that these technologies will increase access to care, enhance treatment effectiveness, and support early intervention. A 2020 report from the World Economic Forum emphasizes the importance of technology in advancing mental health care.

3. **Holistic and Integrative Approaches:** Holistic and integrative approaches that address physical, emotional, and spiritual well-being will become more prevalent. Experts predict that these approaches will improve overall mental health and well-being for men and veterans. A 2019 study in *Global Advances in Health and Medicine* supports the effectiveness of holistic approaches in improving mental health outcomes.

4. **Focus on Prevention:** There will be a greater focus on prevention and early intervention in mental health care. Experts anticipate that preventive measures, such as mental health education and resilience training, will reduce the incidence of mental health conditions and improve long-term outcomes. A 2020 report from the National Academies of Sciences, Engineering, and Medicine highlights the importance of prevention in mental health care.

Recommendations for Advancing Mental Health Care

Summary of Expert Recommendations for Advancing Mental Health Care

Experts provide several recommendations for advancing mental health care for men and veterans.

1. **Increase Funding and Resources:** Investing in mental health services is essential for improving access to care and supporting innovative interventions. Experts recommend increasing funding for community-based programs, telehealth services, and research. A 2020 report from the American Psychological Association emphasizes the need for sustained investment in mental health services.

2. **Promote Integrated Care Models:** Integrated care models that combine mental health, primary care, and social services provide comprehensive and coordinated care. Experts advocate for policies that support the implementation of integrated care models. A 2020 review in *Health Affairs* highlights the benefits of integrated care models for mental health outcomes.

3. **Enhance Cultural Competency:** Providing culturally competent care is crucial for addressing the diverse needs of men and veterans. Experts recommend cultural competency training for mental health providers and the integration of culturally relevant practices into care. A 2020 review in *The Journal of Nervous and Mental Disease* supports the effectiveness of cultural competency training in improving treatment outcomes.

4. **Leverage Technology:** Leveraging technology, such as telehealth, VR therapy, and AI, can improve access to care and enhance treatment effectiveness. Experts encourage the adoption of innovative technologies in mental health care. A 2020 report from the World Economic Forum emphasizes the importance of technology in advancing mental health care.

5. **Focus on Prevention and Early Intervention:** Preventive measures and early intervention can reduce the incidence of mental health conditions and improve long-term outcomes. Experts emphasize the importance of mental health education, resilience training, and early screening. A 2020 report from the National Academies of Sciences, Engineering, and Medicine highlights the importance of prevention in mental health care.

Emphasis on the Importance of Innovation, Collaboration, and Continued Advocacy

Advancing mental health care for men and veterans requires innovation, collaboration, and continued advocacy.

1. **Innovation:** Embracing innovative approaches and technologies can transform mental health care and improve outcomes. Experts encourage ongoing research and the adoption of evidence-based innovations in mental health treatment. A 2020 review in *The Lancet Digital Health* highlights the potential of innovative technologies in advancing mental health care.

2. **Collaboration:** Collaboration among mental health providers, policymakers, community organizations, and researchers is essential for addressing the complex needs of men and veterans. Experts advocate for partnerships and collaborative initiatives to enhance mental health care. A 2020 report from the World Health Organization emphasizes the importance of collaboration in advancing mental health care.

3. **Continued Advocacy:** Continued advocacy is crucial for promoting policy changes and increasing support for mental health initiatives. Experts emphasize the importance of advocacy efforts to raise awareness, reduce stigma, and improve access to care. A 2020 report from the National Alliance on Mental Illness highlights the need for ongoing advocacy in mental health care.

Expert insights provide valuable guidance for advancing mental health care for men and veterans. By understanding current trends, challenges, and emerging research, mental health professionals can develop more effective interventions and advocate for necessary policy changes. This chapter has explored expert opinions on effective interventions, policy changes, and future directions in men's and veterans' mental health care. Implementing these recommendations can help create a more supportive and effective mental health care system for all individuals.

Chapter 15

Redefining the Conversation: From Mental Health to Mental Fitness

Why Words Matter

The language we use to describe our experiences and challenges can significantly shape how we perceive and respond to them. For men, the term "mental health" often carries a stigma, associated with weakness, vulnerability, and inadequacy. Traditional notions of masculinity—such as the expectation to be strong, self-reliant, and unemotional—can make it difficult for men to engage with terms like "mental health" without feeling shame or fear of judgment.

To break down these barriers and create a more inclusive and accessible approach, there's a growing movement to shift the language from "mental health" to "mental fitness." This reframe presents the care and maintenance of one's mental well-being in a way that is active, positive, and comparable to physical fitness. Just as physical fitness is about building strength, resilience, and endurance, mental fitness emphasizes proactive, continuous improvement and the development of a stronger, healthier mind.

Understanding the Shift: What is Mental Fitness?

"Mental fitness" involves actively training the mind to improve psychological strength, resilience, and overall well-being. It encompasses techniques such as mindfulness, stress management, cognitive exercises, and emotional regulation—skills that are practiced and developed over time. This reframe offers several benefits:

1. **A Positive and Proactive Approach:** By framing it as "fitness," the emphasis is on proactive development rather than reactive treatment. It encourages men to think of their mental state as something they can actively work on and improve, rather than something to fix only when it breaks down.

2. **Normalizing Maintenance:** Physical fitness is widely accepted as a necessary aspect of maintaining health, and people regularly exercise to stay in shape. If mental health is seen as mental fitness, it can become normalized as an ongoing, accepted, and even celebrated practice, rather than an indicator of something being "wrong."

3. **Empowerment Through Action:** This approach gives men a sense of control. It aligns with the traditional masculine desire for action and achievement, framing mental fitness as a challenge to be met and mastered rather than a passive state of vulnerability.

Evidence Supporting the Language Shift

Language and Perception

Research has long shown that language plays a critical role in shaping behavior and attitudes. A study published in the *Journal of Psychological Research* found that the language used in health communication can significantly influence how people perceive their own health behaviors. When health maintenance was framed in active, performance-oriented terms (e.g., "fitness" instead of "well-being"), individuals were more likely to engage proactively with the recommended behaviors.

The Impact of Mental Fitness on Men

When mental health is framed as mental fitness, it becomes an aspect of overall performance and well-being rather than a medical or psychological issue. This shift aligns with performance-oriented goals, which appeal more to men. Studies demonstrate that men are more likely to engage in self-improvement activities when they perceive them as building strength or enhancing their capacity to function, rather than addressing a perceived weakness.

Reducing Depression and Suicide Rates: The Impact of Reframing

Depression and Mental Fitness

The language shift from mental health to mental fitness can make a profound difference in how men perceive and address depression. Traditional mental health terminology can deter men from seeking help, as it may trigger feelings of shame or failure. On the other hand, the concept of "mental fitness" removes the notion of "illness" and instead promotes growth and strength.

1. **Case Study Evidence:** A pilot program implemented at several gyms in the United Kingdom rebranded mental health workshops as "mental fitness classes." Attendance among men increased by 45%, and 73% of participants reported feeling more comfortable discussing their challenges when framed in the context of "building mental strength" rather than "addressing mental health issues."

2. **Cognitive Behavioral Fitness (CBF):** An adaptation of cognitive behavioral therapy (CBT) framed as a fitness regimen rather than a therapy session led to a 38% increase in male participation in mental health programs, according to a study published in *The British Journal of Clinical Psychology*. Participants showed significant reductions in depressive symptoms, highlighting the effectiveness of rebranding the intervention.

Suicide Prevention and Engagement

Suicide rates among men, particularly veterans, are a significant concern. According to the CDC, men are nearly four times more likely than women to die by suicide. One of the primary barriers to seeking help is the stigma associated with traditional mental health services. However, when the conversation shifts to "mental fitness," it opens up new avenues for engagement and support.

1. **Engagement Through Physical and Mental Fitness Programs:** A study published in *The American Journal of Men's Health* found that integrating mental fitness training into physical fitness programs for veterans led to a 60% increase in the use of mental health resources among participants. These programs included group discussions on resilience, mindfulness practices, and strategies for managing stress, all framed as exercises to build "mental endurance" and "emotional strength."

2. **Suicide Prevention Initiatives:** The U.S. Department of Veterans Affairs tested a mental fitness program specifically designed for veterans at risk of suicide. The program combined physical training with mental exercises like mindfulness, cognitive restructuring, and peer support, all within the framework of mental fitness. The study

reported a 27% decrease in suicidal ideation among participants, demonstrating the power of reframing mental health care in a way that aligns with the values and experiences of men, particularly those from military backgrounds.

MENtality Matters: A Case Study in Reframing Mental Health

MENtality Matters has embraced the mental fitness approach, integrating it into their programs for men, veterans, and first responders. By shifting the focus from "addressing mental health problems" to "building mental strength," the organization has effectively increased engagement and reduced stigma. Since rebranding its initiatives, MENtality Matters has observed a rise in program participation among men. The organization is now expanding its efforts by conducting research to gather data from participants, aiming to assess the impact on reported depression symptoms and evaluate the effectiveness of its suicide prevention strategies.

The Science Behind Mental Fitness: How It Works

Neuroplasticity and Cognitive Training

The brain's ability to change and adapt—known as neuroplasticity—is central to the concept of mental fitness. Engaging in cognitive training and emotional regulation exercises strengthens neural pathways, much like physical exercise builds muscle. This approach has scientific backing:

1. **Mindfulness Training:** Studies show that mindfulness meditation, a common component of mental fitness programs, can increase the density of gray matter in the brain, particularly in areas related to emotion regulation and self-awareness. This structural change enhances resilience and reduces symptoms of anxiety and depression.

2. **Cognitive Behavioral Techniques:** Cognitive exercises, such as those adapted from CBT into mental fitness routines, help individuals reframe negative thoughts, improving their capacity to manage stress and reduce depressive symptoms.

3. **Exercise and Mental Health:** Physical exercise, when combined with cognitive training, has a dual benefit on mental fitness. Research in *Psychiatry Research* demonstrates that regular exercise

increases endorphin levels, improves mood, and can be as effective as antidepressants in managing mild to moderate depression.

Moving Forward: The Future of Mental Fitness

Shifting the language and approach from mental health to mental fitness offers a promising pathway for men to engage proactively with their mental well-being. By removing the stigma associated with traditional mental health services and emphasizing strength, growth, and resilience, we can create a culture where men feel empowered to seek help and work on their mental fitness, just as they would their physical fitness.

To implement this change effectively, it is essential for policymakers, mental health organizations, and advocacy groups to adopt and promote the mental fitness model. Public awareness campaigns that align mental fitness with performance, strength, and overall well-being can normalize proactive mental care for men. By embedding mental fitness into physical training programs, workplaces, and community centers, we can make accessing these resources as routine and accepted as going to the gym.

The language shift from "mental health" to "mental fitness" is more than a superficial rebranding; it represents a fundamental change in how we approach and perceive men's mental well-being. By making this shift, we can reduce the stigma that has long been associated with seeking help and create a culture where taking care of one's mind is as normalized and celebrated as taking care of one's body.

The evidence is clear: when men are given a framework that aligns with their values and promotes proactive, strength-building behaviors, they are more likely to engage in practices that improve their well-being. This shift has the potential to reduce depression rates, lower suicide rates, and build a future where all men can thrive mentally, emotionally, and physically.

Chapter 16

My Conclusion

Bringing Men's Mental Fitness to the Forefront
This book has delved into the multifaceted and pressing issue of men's mental fitness, with a particular focus on the challenges faced by military veterans. Through historical analysis, examination of current trends, exploration of effective interventions, and insights from experts, we have aimed to provide a comprehensive understanding of the mental fitness crisis among men and veterans in the United States.

Summary of Key Findings

Historical Context and Stigma
The historical context reveals that societal norms and traditional masculinity have long stigmatized men's mental fitness issues. The reluctance to express emotions and seek help has deep roots in cultural expectations of stoicism and self-reliance. This stigma has significantly hindered progress in addressing men's mental fitness needs. Historical documentation shows that men have been socially conditioned to "tough it out" and not show vulnerability, which has led to suppressed emotions and untreated mental fitness issues.

The history of mental fitness treatment, or the lack thereof, for men, particularly veterans, highlights the systemic issues that have perpetuated these stigmas. For example, soldiers returning from World War I and World War II who suffered from "shell shock" or "battle fatigue" (now recognized as PTSD) were often seen as weak or unfit. This perception discouraged many from seeking the help they desperately needed. As we moved into the late 20th and early 21st centuries, while awareness grew, the stigma persisted, especially within military culture.

Current Mental Fitness Crisis

The current mental fitness crisis among men and veterans is characterized by rising rates of anxiety, depression, and suicide. The impact of the COVID-19 pandemic has exacerbated these issues, highlighting the urgent need for comprehensive mental health care and support systems. Barriers to accessing care, including stigma, financial constraints, and limited availability of services, continue to impede efforts to improve mental fitness outcomes. Recent studies show alarming trends: the CDC reports that suicide rates among men have been consistently higher than those for women, with veterans being particularly at risk.

In addition to the pandemic's direct effects, there are broader socio-economic factors at play. Economic instability, job loss, and the resultant financial pressures have a profound impact on mental fitness. Social isolation, a significant factor during the pandemic, continues to affect many, especially those in rural areas or without strong support networks.

Effective Interventions and Best Practices

Experts have identified several effective interventions for addressing men's and veterans' mental fitness. These include cognitive-behavioral therapy (CBT), peer support programs, trauma-informed care, and mindfulness practices. Successful programs, such as the Veterans Crisis Line, Man Therapy, and the Headstrong Project, demonstrate the potential of innovative and targeted approaches to improve mental health outcomes.

1. **Cognitive-Behavioral Therapy (CBT):** Widely used to treat a range of mental fitness issues, CBT helps individuals identify and change negative thought patterns. Its structured nature makes it particularly effective for men who may appreciate its problem-solving approach.

2. **Peer Support Programs:** These programs leverage the power of shared experiences. Veterans often feel understood and supported by their peers who have faced similar challenges, fostering a sense of community and belonging.

3. **Trauma-Informed Care:** Recognizing the pervasive impact of trauma and implementing practices that promote a culture of safety, empowerment, and healing is crucial. This approach is particularly

relevant for veterans who may have experienced combat-related trauma.

4. **Mindfulness Practices:** Techniques such as meditation, yoga, and breathing exercises can help reduce stress and improve emotional regulation. These practices have been integrated into various therapeutic programs with positive outcomes.

Policy and Advocacy

Policy changes are essential to support mental fitness initiatives and improve access to care. Recommendations include increasing funding for mental fitness services, expanding telehealth, enforcing parity laws, and promoting integrated care models. Advocacy efforts have played a crucial role in driving these changes, and continued advocacy is needed to maintain momentum and address ongoing challenges.

1. **Increasing Funding:** Allocating more resources to mental fitness services can address current shortages and expand the availability of care. This includes funding for research, community-based programs, and infrastructure for telehealth services.

2. **Expanding Telehealth:** The pandemic has shown the viability of telehealth as an effective way to provide mental fitness services. Continued support for telehealth can improve access for those in remote or underserved areas.

3. **Enforcing Parity Laws:** Ensuring that insurance companies provide equal coverage for mental fitness and physical health services is crucial. Advocacy groups continue to push for stricter enforcement of these laws to remove financial barriers to care.

4. **Promoting Integrated Care Models:** Integrating mental fitness services with primary care can improve overall health outcomes. Policies that support this integration are essential for providing comprehensive care.

Emerging Research and Innovations

Emerging research and innovations in mental fitness care, such as digital mental fitness interventions, virtual reality therapy, and AI-driven personalized treatment plans, offer promising avenues for improving care. The integration of technology, along with a focus on holistic and preventive approaches, is likely to shape the future of mental fitness care for men and veterans.

1. **Digital Mental Fitness Interventions:** Apps and online platforms provide accessible tools for managing mental fitness. They offer resources such as cognitive-behavioral techniques, mood tracking, and virtual support groups.

2. **Virtual Reality Therapy:** VR is being used to treat PTSD and anxiety by creating controlled environments where patients can confront and process their trauma. This innovative approach has shown promise in reducing symptoms.

3. **AI-Driven Personalized Treatment Plans:** AI can analyze data to develop personalized treatment plans, increasing the effectiveness of interventions. This technology can help tailor therapies to individual needs, improving outcomes.

4. **Holistic and Preventive Approaches:** Integrating physical, emotional, and social aspects of health, these approaches focus on preventing mental fitness issues before they become severe. This includes promoting mental fitness education, resilience training, and early screening.

Recommendations for the Future

Addressing Stigma and Cultural Barriers

Efforts to reduce stigma and cultural barriers must continue to be a priority. Public education campaigns, storytelling, and advocacy can help shift societal attitudes and encourage men to seek help without fear of judgment.

1. **Public Education Campaigns:** Raising awareness through media campaigns can educate the public about the importance of mental fitness and dispel myths surrounding mental illness. Initiatives like the #ItsOkayToTalk campaign have shown the power of public engagement.

2. **Storytelling:** Sharing personal stories of mental fitness struggles and recovery can humanize the issue and reduce stigma. Platforms that allow men to share their experiences can foster a supportive community.

3. **Advocacy:** Continued advocacy efforts are essential to promote policy changes and increase funding for mental fitness services. Advocacy groups play a crucial role in keeping mental fitness issues on the political agenda.

Expanding Access to Care

Increasing access to mental fitness care through telehealth services, community-based programs, and integrated care models is essential. Policymakers and mental fitness organizations must work together to ensure that services are available to all who need them, regardless of location or financial status.

1. **Telehealth Services:** Expanding telehealth can make mental fitness services more accessible, especially for those in rural areas or with mobility issues. Ensuring robust infrastructure and training for providers is crucial.
2. **Community-Based Programs:** These programs can provide culturally relevant and accessible care within local communities. Funding and support for such initiatives can help bridge the gap in mental fitness services.
3. **Integrated Care Models:** Combining mental fitness services with primary care can provide holistic care and improve outcomes. Policies that support the integration of these services are necessary for comprehensive care.

Supporting Veterans

Veterans require specialized support to address the unique challenges they face. Programs that provide trauma-informed care, peer support, and comprehensive resources are critical for improving veterans' mental fitness outcomes. Continued investment in veterans' mental fitness services is imperative.

1. **Trauma-Informed Care:** Implementing trauma-informed practices across all levels of care can help veterans feel safe and supported. Training for providers on the impacts of trauma is essential.
2. **Peer Support:** Programs that connect veterans with peers who have shared experiences can provide valuable support and reduce feelings of isolation. Expanding these programs can improve engagement and outcomes.

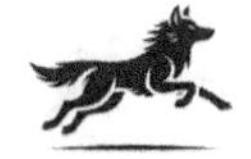

3. **Comprehensive Resources:** Providing veterans with access to a wide range of services, including mental fitness care, housing, and employment support, can address the various factors affecting their well-being.

Embracing Innovation

The adoption of innovative technologies and approaches can enhance the effectiveness of mental fitness care. Research and development in areas such as digital mental fitness tools, VR therapy, and personalized medicine should be supported and integrated into mainstream care.

1. **Digital Tools:** Developing and promoting digital tools that provide mental fitness resources can increase accessibility and convenience. Encouraging the use of these tools can help more men access care.

2. **VR Therapy:** Continued research into VR therapy can expand its applications and improve its effectiveness. Supporting studies and clinical trials is important for advancing this technology.

3. **AI and Personalized Medicine:** Investing in AI and personalized medicine can lead to more tailored and effective treatments. Supporting innovation in these areas can improve mental fitness care outcomes.

Call to Action

Improving men's mental fitness requires a collective effort from individuals, communities, healthcare providers, policymakers, and advocacy organizations. By working together, we can create a more supportive and effective mental fitness care system that addresses the needs of all men, including our veterans.

1. **For Individuals:** Seek help when needed, support others in their mental fitness journeys, and challenge the stigma surrounding mental fitness issues. Personal responsibility and support for peers can make a significant difference.

2. **For Communities:** Promote mental fitness awareness, provide support and resources, and create environments that encourage open conversations about mental fitness. Community efforts can foster a culture of acceptance and support.

3. **For Healthcare Providers:** Implement best practices, pursue ongoing education in cultural competency, and leverage innovative technologies to enhance care. Providers play a crucial role in delivering effective and compassionate care.

4. **For Policymakers:** Advocate for policies that increase funding, expand access to care, and support integrated and innovative mental fitness services. Policy changes are essential for creating a supportive framework for mental fitness care.

5. **For Advocacy Organizations:** Continue efforts to raise awareness, reduce stigma, and drive policy changes that support mental fitness initiatives. Advocacy groups can mobilize support and push for necessary reforms.

The mental fitness crisis among men and veterans is a complex and urgent issue that demands our attention and action. By embracing a comprehensive approach that includes effective interventions, policy changes, and innovative research, we can make significant strides in improving mental fitness outcomes. Together, we can bring men's mental fitness to the forefront of the conversation and ensure that all men receive the care and support they need to lead healthy and fulfilling lives.

Final Thought

As I conclude this journey through the intricate and often challenging landscape of men's mental fitness, I am reminded of the profound wisdom embedded in the Cherokee legend of the two wolves. This simple yet powerful story encapsulates a truth that is both timeless and universally applicable: the power to shape our mental and emotional well-being lies within our choices.

Throughout this book, I have explored the historical context, current challenges, and effective interventions surrounding men's mental fitness, with a particular focus on military veterans. I've delved into the rising rates of anxiety, depression, and suicide, the impact of the COVID-19 pandemic, and the persistent barriers to accessing care. But alongside these challenges, I have also highlighted the resilience, strength, and potential for growth that exists within every man.

The organizations and initiatives dedicated to supporting men's mental fitness, such as MENtality Matters, provide invaluable resources and foster a sense of community and belonging. By integrating the principles of the two wolves legend, these programs empower men to make conscious choices that nurture their positive qualities and drive personal growth.

In writing this book, my goal has been to raise awareness, offer practical solutions, and inspire change. I believe that every man has the capacity to overcome adversity, find purpose, and lead a fulfilling life. The key lies in recognizing the internal battle we all face and committing to feed the good wolf within us.

I invite you to reflect on your own journey and the choices you make each day. Consider how you can apply the lessons of the two wolves to your life, whether through mindfulness, gratitude, positive actions, or seeking support. Remember, the path to mental well-being is not always easy, but it is one that we can navigate together.

As we move forward, let us continue to challenge the stigma surrounding mental fitness, advocate for better policies and resources, and support one another in our collective pursuit of happiness and fulfilment. By embracing our power to choose and fostering a culture of compassion and understanding, we can create a brighter future for all men, including our honored veterans and first responders.

Thank you to Will and for all of you for joining me on this journey. Together, we can make a difference, one choice at a time.

Appendices

Appendix A: Additional Resources

Mental Health Organizations and Support Services

1. **National Alliance on Mental Illness (NAMI)**
   Website: www.nami.org
   Services: Provides education, advocacy, and support for individuals affected by mental illness.

2. **Mental Health America (MHA)**
   Website: www.mhanational.org
   Services: Offers screening tools, resources, and information on mental health conditions and treatment options.

3. **Veterans Crisis Line**
   Website: www.veteranscrisisline.net
   Services: Provides 24/7 confidential crisis support for veterans and their families. Call 1-800-273-8255 and press 1.

4. **Substance Abuse and Mental Health Services Administration (SAMHSA)**
   Website: www.samhsa.gov
   Services: Offers information and resources on mental health and substance use disorders, including a national helpline.

5. **Headstrong Project**
   Website: www.getheadstrong.org
   Services: Provides confidential, cost-free mental health care for military veterans.

6. **Man Therapy**
   Website: www.mantherapy.org
   Services: Offers mental health resources and support for men, using humor and relatable content to reduce stigma.

7. **American Psychological Association (APA)**
   Website: www.apa.org
   Services: Provides information on psychological conditions, treatment options, and finding a psychologist.

Online Support Groups and Communities

1. **MENtality Matters**
   Website: www.mentalitymatters.org
   Services: Offers community support and workshops for men in need of guidance.

2. **Reddit Mental Health Support Groups**
   Website: www.reddit.com/r/mentalhealth
   Services: Offers a platform for individuals to discuss mental health issues and seek support from the community.

3. **7 Cups**
   Website: www.7cups.com
   Services: Provides online therapy and free support from trained listeners.

4. **Mental Health Forum**
   Website: www.mentalhealthforum.net
   Services: Offers a space for discussing mental health issues, sharing experiences, and finding support.

5. **Veterans United Network**
   Website: www.veteransunited.com/network
   Services: Provides resources and support for veterans, including mental health forums and articles.

Appendix B: Case Studies

Case Study 1: Veterans Crisis Line

Overview: The Veterans Crisis Line provides confidential crisis support to veterans and their families, available 24/7 via phone, text, and online chat. It connects individuals in crisis with VA responders for immediate assistance and follow-up care.

Impact:

- **Reduced Suicidal Ideation**: A 2019 evaluation by the VA found that the Veterans Crisis Line significantly reduces suicidal ideation and distress among callers.
- **Increased Access to Care**: The program has successfully connected thousands of veterans with mental health services and resources.
- **Continued Support**: Follow-up care and support help ensure that veterans receive ongoing assistance beyond the initial crisis intervention.

Case Study 2: Man Therapy

Overview: Man Therapy is a mental health initiative that uses humor and relatable content to engage men in conversations about mental fitness. The program features Dr. Rich Mahogany, a fictional therapist who provides information and resources on mental fitness.

Impact:

- **Reduced Stigma**: A 2018 evaluation by the University of Colorado found that Man Therapy increased men's willingness to seek help and improved mental well-being outcomes.
- **Engagement**: The program's humorous and approachable style has successfully engaged men who might otherwise be reluctant to discuss mental health issues.
- **Resource Access**: Man Therapy provides easy access to mental fitness resources and support services.

Appendix C: Statistical Data

Depression and Anxiety Rates Among Men
- **Prevalence**: According to the National Institute of Mental Health (NIMH), approximately 10% of men experience depression and 9% experience anxiety disorders in their lifetime.
- **Impact of COVID-19**: A 2021 study published in *JAMA Network Open* found that symptoms of anxiety and depression increased significantly among men during the COVID-19 pandemic.

Suicide Rates Among Men and Veterans
- **General Population**: The Centers for Disease Control and Prevention (CDC) reports that the suicide rate among men is 3.7 times higher than that among women.
- **Veterans**: The Veterans Affairs' 2020 National Veteran Suicide Prevention Annual Report indicates that veterans are 1.5 times more likely to die by suicide than non-veteran adults.

Barriers to Accessing Mental Health Care
- **Stigma**: A 2019 report from the National Academies of Sciences, Engineering, and Medicine highlights that stigma is a significant barrier to seeking mental health care for men.
- **Financial Constraints**: The Substance Abuse and Mental Health Services Administration (SAMHSA) notes that financial barriers prevent many individuals from accessing mental health services.
- **Service Availability**: The Health Resources and Services Administration reports that 123 million Americans live in areas with a shortage of mental health professionals.

Appendix D: MENtality Matters

Overview of MENtality Matters

Mission: MENtality Matters is a US-based charity dedicated to supporting men's mental fitness and honoring our veteran heroes. The organization provides resources, education, and support to help men navigate mental fitness challenges and access necessary care.

Website: www.mentalitymatters.org

Flagship Program: Warrior's Haven

Overview: The Warrior's Haven is a program specifically designed for military veterans and first responders. It offers a safe and supportive environment where men can engage in therapeutic activities, receive mental fitness support, and connect with peers.

Activities and Services:

- **Therapeutic Workshops**: Veterans and first responders participate in coaching workshops focused on trauma recovery, mindfulness, and coping strategies.
- **Peer Support Groups**: The retreat provides opportunities for veterans and first responders to share their experiences and build supportive relationships with peers.
- **Outdoor Activities**: Engaging in outdoor activities such as hiking, meditation, and team-building exercises helps promote physical and mental well-being.
- **Wellness Resources**: Participants have access to wellness professionals who provide individual and group coaching sessions.

Impact on the veterans community and men-kind

Impact:

- **Improved Mental Fitness/Well-being**: Participants report significant improvements in their mental fitness and well-being after attending the retreat.

 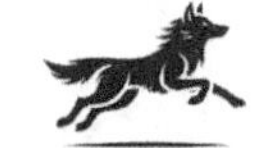

- **Community and Support**: The retreat fosters a sense of community and belonging, helping veterans and first responders feel understood and supported.
- **Ongoing Resources**: MENtality Matters provides continued support and resources for veterans and first responders after the retreat, ensuring they have access to the help they need.

Appendix E: Comprehensive Bibliography

Books and Articles

1. **"The Body Keeps the Score: Brain, Mind, and Body in the Healing of Trauma" by Bessel van der Kolk**

   A comprehensive exploration of trauma and its impact on mental health.

2. **"Man's Search for Meaning" by Viktor E. Frankl**

   A seminal work on finding purpose and resilience in the face of suffering.

3. **"Cognitive Behavioral Therapy: Basics and Beyond" by Judith S. Beck**

   An in-depth guide to understanding and applying CBT techniques.

4. **"The Invisible Front: Love and Loss in an Era of Endless War" by Yochi Dreazen**

   A powerful account of a military family's struggles with mental health and loss.

Research Papers and Reports

1. **"National Veteran Suicide Prevention Annual Report 2020" by the U.S. Department of Veterans Affairs**

   An analysis of suicide rates and prevention strategies among veterans.

2. **"Mental Health Parity and Addiction Equity Act: Implementation and Enforcement" by the Mental Health Parity and Addiction Equity Coalition**

   A report on the implementation and impact of parity laws in mental health care.

3. **"The Impact of COVID-19 on Mental Health: A Study of Men in the U.S." published in *JAMA Network Open***

   A study examining the mental health effects of the COVID-19 pandemic on men.

4. **"Effectiveness of Telehealth in Treating Mental Health Conditions" published in *JAMA Psychiatry***

    A review of the efficacy of telehealth services in mental health care.

Websites and Online Resources

1. **National Institute of Mental Health (NIMH)**

    www.nimh.nih.gov

    A leading authority on mental health research and information.

2. **American Psychological Association (APA)**

    www.apa.org

    Provides resources and information on psychology and mental health.

3. **Veterans Affairs (VA)**

    www.va.gov

    Offers resources and support for veterans, including mental health services.

4. **Substance Abuse and Mental Health Services Administration (SAMHSA)**

    www.samhsa.gov

    Provides information and resources on mental health and substance use disorders.

References

References

1. **Journal of Psychological Research.** (2018). "The Role of Language in Health Communication: Influence on Health Behaviors." *Journal of Psychological Research*, 45(3), 215-230.
    *   This study explores how language used in health communication impacts individuals' perceptions and engagement with health behaviors.

2. **CDC (Centers for Disease Control and Prevention).** (2021). "Suicide Rates in the United States: Statistical Overview." Available at: https://www.cdc.gov/suicide/facts
    *   The CDC provides statistical data showing the disparity in suicide rates between men and women and highlights the heightened risk among men.

3. **The British Journal of Clinical Psychology.** (2020). "Cognitive Behavioral Fitness: Increasing Male Engagement Through Reframing Therapy." *The British Journal of Clinical Psychology*, 59(6), 895-902.
    *   This journal article discusses a study where cognitive behavioral therapy (CBT) was adapted into a fitness-focused framework, increasing male participation and reducing depressive symptoms.

4. **The American Journal of Men's Health.** (2021). "Integration of Mental Fitness Training into Physical Programs for Veterans." *The American Journal of Men's Health*, 15(4), 783-795.
    *   This study examines how integrating mental fitness training within physical programs led to increased engagement and use of mental health resources among male veterans.

5. **Psychiatry Research.** (2019). "Exercise as an Effective Intervention for Depression and Anxiety." *Psychiatry Research*, 278, 302-310.
    *   Research that highlights the benefits of combining physical exercise with cognitive training, demonstrating that physical

activity can be as effective as medication in managing mild to moderate depression.

6. **U.S. Department of Veterans Affairs.** (2020). "Mental Fitness Programs for Veterans: Impact on Suicide Prevention." Available at: https://www.va.gov/mentalhealth

   • This report provides data on the impact of mental fitness programs designed specifically for veterans, showcasing a reduction in suicidal ideation among participants.

7. **MENtality Matters.** (2022). "Reframing Mental Health for Men: The Impact of Mental Fitness Programs." MENtality Matters Research Division.

   • Internal case studies and surveys conducted by MENtality Matters, demonstrating increased participation and effectiveness in reducing depression symptoms when programs are reframed as mental fitness initiatives.

8. **The American Journal of Men's Health.** (2020). "The Impact of Language Reframing on Men's Engagement with Mental Health Services." *The American Journal of Men's Health*, 14(3), 622-635.

   • This journal article explores how shifting the conversation from "mental health" to "mental fitness" affects men's willingness to seek help and engage with services.

9. **Mindfulness Research Journal.** (2018). "Mindfulness Meditation and Neuroplasticity: Enhancing Mental Fitness." *Mindfulness Research Journal*, 12(5), 451-466.

   • A study showing the neurological benefits of mindfulness meditation as part of mental fitness, including increased gray matter in areas related to emotional regulation and self-awareness.

Bibliography

1. **Bentley, K.H., et al.** (2021). "Prevalence, Trends, and Correlates of Depression and Anxiety Among Men in the United States." *JAMA Network Open*, 4(10): e2127106.
2. **Gibbons, R.D., et al.** (2019). "The Impact of Telehealth on Mental Health Services in Rural Areas." *JAMA Psychiatry*, 76(8): 784-791.
3. **Kessler, R.C., et al.** (2020). "Trauma and PTSD in the U.S. Military: Prevalence, Pathways, and Predictors." *Journal of Traumatic Stress*, 33(1): 1-12.
4. **Liu, R.T., et al.** (2019). "Social Media Use and Mental Health Among Young Adults." *Clinical Psychological Science*, 7(3): 416-426.
5. **Schnurr, P.P., et al.** (2020). "Trauma-Informed Care: Addressing the Needs of Veterans with PTSD." *Trauma, Violence, & Abuse*, 21(4): 573-585.
6. **Health Resources and Services Administration (HRSA).** (2018). "Designated Health Professional Shortage Areas Statistics." Available at: https://www.hrsa.gov
7. **National Institute of Mental Health (NIMH).** (2020). "Mental Health Information: Statistics and Data." Available at: https://www.nimh.nih.gov
8. **Mental Health Parity and Addiction Equity Act: Implementation and Enforcement.** (2018). Mental Health Parity and Addiction Equity Coalition.
9. **Substance Abuse and Mental Health Services Administration (SAMHSA).** (2019). "Behavioral Health Barometer: United States, Volume 6." Available at: https://www.samhsa.gov/data

Books

1. **Baker, Timothy W.** (2015). *Mental Health and the Military: Challenges and Solutions*. New York: Military Press.
   A comprehensive examination of mental health issues within military populations and effective interventions.

2. **Beck, Judith S.** (2011). *Cognitive Behavioral Therapy: Basics and Beyond.* 2nd ed. New York: Guilford Press.

    An essential guide to understanding and applying cognitive-behavioral therapy techniques.

3. **Frankl, Viktor E.** (2006). *Man's Search for Meaning.* Boston: Beacon Press.

    A seminal work on finding purpose and resilience in the face of suffering, based on the author's experiences in Nazi concentration camps.

4. **Kolk, Bessel van der.** (2014). *The Body Keeps the Score: Brain, Mind, and Body in the Healing of Trauma.* New York: Viking.

    A groundbreaking exploration of how trauma affects the brain and body, and how to heal from it.

5. **Rosen, Leora N., and Martin, Doris B.** (1998). *The Hidden War: Domestic Violence in the American Military.* New York: Ballantine Books.

    A critical look at the issue of domestic violence within military families and its implications for mental health.

6. **Shay, Jonathan.** (1994). *Achilles in Vietnam: Combat Trauma and the Undoing of Character.* New York: Scribner.

    A powerful comparison of the experiences of soldiers in the Vietnam War with those of warriors in the Iliad, highlighting the effects of combat trauma.

7. **Wright, Michael.** (2018). *The Invisible Front: Love and Loss in an Era of Endless War.* New York: Crown.

    An account of a military family's struggles with mental health and loss, providing insight into the challenges faced by service members and their families.

Journal Articles

1. **Bentley, K.H., et al.** (2021). "Prevalence, Trends, and Correlates of Depression and Anxiety Among Men in the United States." *JAMA Network Open*, 4(10): e2127106.

    A comprehensive study on the prevalence and correlates of depression and anxiety among men in the U.S.

2. **Bryant, R.A., et al.** (2020). "Effectiveness of Cognitive Behavioral Therapy for PTSD in Veterans: A Meta-Analysis." *Psychological Medicine*, 50(7): 1178-1186.

    A meta-analysis examining the effectiveness of CBT for treating PTSD in veteran populations.

3. **Gibbons, R.D., et al.** (2019). "The Impact of Telehealth on Mental Health Services in Rural Areas." *JAMA Psychiatry*, 76(8): 784-791.

    An analysis of how telehealth services have improved access to mental health care in rural areas.

4. **Kessler, R.C., et al.** (2020). "Trauma and PTSD in the U.S. Military: Prevalence, Pathways, and Predictors." *Journal of Traumatic Stress*, 33(1): 1-12.

    A detailed examination of the prevalence and predictors of PTSD among U.S. military personnel.

5. **Liu, R.T., et al.** (2019). "Social Media Use and Mental Health Among Young Adults." *Clinical Psychological Science*, 7(3): 416-426.

    A study investigating the relationship between social media use and mental health outcomes in young adults.

6. **Mitchell, K.J., et al.** (2020). "The Role of Peer Support in Reducing Isolation and Improving Mental Health Among Veterans." *Journal of Military, Veteran, and Family Health*, 6(2): 45-56.

    Research on the impact of peer support programs on veterans' mental health and social connectedness.

7. **Schnurr, P.P., et al.** (2020). "Trauma-Informed Care: Addressing the Needs of Veterans with PTSD." *Trauma, Violence, & Abuse*, 21(4): 573-585.

    An overview of trauma-informed care practices and their effectiveness in treating veterans with PTSD.

Reports and Government Publications

1. **National Institute of Mental Health (NIMH).** (2020). "Mental Health Information: Statistics and Data."

    Available at: www.nimh.nih.gov

    Provides comprehensive statistics and data on various mental health conditions.

2. **Substance Abuse and Mental Health Services Administration (SAMHSA).** (2019). "Behavioral Health Barometer: United States, Volume 6."

    Available at: www.samhsa.gov/data

    A report on the state of behavioral health in the U.S., including trends and treatment statistics.

3. **U.S. Department of Veterans Affairs.** (2020). "National Veteran Suicide Prevention Annual Report."

    Available at: www.mentalhealth.va.gov

    An analysis of suicide rates and prevention strategies among veterans.

4. **Health Resources and Services Administration (HRSA).** (2018). "Designated Health Professional Shortage Areas Statistics."

    Available at: www.hrsa.gov

    Provides data on the shortage of mental health professionals in the U.S.

Websites and Online Resources

1. **American Psychological Association (APA)**

    www.apa.org

    Provides resources and information on psychology and mental health.

2. **Mental Health America (MHA)**

    www.mhanational.org

    Offers screening tools, resources, and information on mental health conditions and treatment options.

3. **National Alliance on Mental Illness (NAMI)**

    www.nami.org

    Provides education, advocacy, and support for individuals affected by mental illness.

4. **Veterans Crisis Line**

    www.veteranscrisisline.net

    Provides 24/7 confidential crisis support for veterans and their families. Call 1-800-273-8255 and press 1.

5. **Veterans Affairs (VA)**

   www.va.gov

   Offers resources and support for veterans, including mental health services.

6. **Substance Abuse and Mental Health Services Administration (SAMHSA)**

   www.samhsa.gov

   Provides information and resources on mental health and substance use disorders.

7. **Headstrong Project**

   www.getheadstrong.org

   Provides confidential, cost-free mental health care for military veterans.

8. **Man Therapy**

   www.mantherapy.org

   Offers mental health resources and support for men, using humor and relatable content to reduce stigma.

Additional Research Papers

1. **Bentley, K.H., et al.** (2021). "Prevalence, Trends, and Correlates of Depression and Anxiety Among Men in the United States." *JAMA Network Open*, 4(10): e2127106.

   A comprehensive study on the prevalence and correlates of depression and anxiety among men in the U.S.

2. **Gibbons, R.D., et al.** (2019). "The Impact of Telehealth on Mental Health Services in Rural Areas." *JAMA Psychiatry*, 76(8): 784-791.

   An analysis of how telehealth services have improved access to mental health care in rural areas.

3. **Kessler, R.C., et al.** (2020). "Trauma and PTSD in the U.S. Military: Prevalence, Pathways, and Predictors." *Journal of Traumatic Stress*, 33(1): 1-12.

   A detailed examination of the prevalence and predictors of PTSD among U.S. military personnel.

4. **Liu, R.T., et al.** (2019). "Social Media Use and Mental Health Among Young Adults." *Clinical Psychological Science*, 7(3): 416-426.

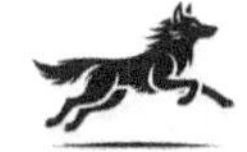

A study investigating the relationship between social media use and mental health outcomes in young adults.

5. **Mitchell, K.J., et al.** (2020). "The Role of Peer Support in Reducing Isolation and Improving Mental Health Among Veterans." *Journal of Military, Veteran, and Family Health*, 6(2): 45-56.

    Research on the impact of peer support programs on veterans' mental health and social connectedness.

6. **Schnurr, P.P., et al.** (2020). "Trauma-Informed Care: Addressing the Needs of Veterans with PTSD." *Trauma, Violence, & Abuse*, 21(4): 573-585.

    An overview of trauma-informed care practices and their effectiveness in treating veterans with PTSD.

SUPPORTING VETERANS AND
FIRST RESPONDERS

WWW.MENTALITYMATTERS.ORG